How to Be Happy, Healthy, Wealthy & Wise

Kent R. McArthur

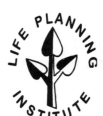

Life Planning Institute, Inc.
P. O. Box 415
Rathdrum, Idaho 83858
Web Site: HappyForLife.com

Published by:
Life Planning Institute, Inc.
P. O. Box 415
Rathdrum, ID 83858
Web Site: HappyForLife.com
Email: LPI@HappyForLife.com

Cover Design & Illustrations by: Nell K. Jehu

Library of Congress Catalog Card No: 98-091289

ISBN: 0-9668078-0-4

Printed and bound by: McNaughton & Gunn, Inc.
Saline, Michigan, USA

"Personality Analysis System Response Sheet" on page 65, Copyright © 1990 Dennis Drew. Reprinted with permission of Drew Software International.

To the

spirit

within you.

Acknowledgements

As with any book there are numerous people to thank for their contributions of time, energy, talent and knowledge: To Bob Ipekdjian for his inspiration and help in defining the scope, focus and tone of the book. To Ellen Meyers for her long discussions and detailed feedback on the early drafts. To David Kohn for his critical thinking and organized editing. To Richard Sisk for his professional review of the manuscript. And, to my soulmate and patient wife, Kathleen who has traveled with me along the path to happiness, good health, wealth and wisdom.

I must also acknowledge the University of California at Berkeley and the Lawrence Berkeley Laboratory. These education and research institutions made it possible for me to take classes and attend workshops that formalized my thinking about life planning. They also made it possible for me to teach classes, counsel and lecture so that I was able to refine the steps of the Life Planning Process.

Finally, my thanks go out to the many students, clients and friends who have allowed me to help them improve the quality of their lives by applying the life planning techniques described in the following pages.

Table of Contents

Foreword

Of course you want to know what qualifies me to show you how to rework your entire life. First, let me tell you about the qualities that I have. Then I'll tell you about my experience. First are my qualities:

- strong analytical abilities—I can examine most systems and situations, diagnose them, and come up with solutions for whatever problems they have.
- a generalist orientation—I have experience in many areas: engineering, business management, computers, college-level teaching, writing and financial planning.
- a strong desire to help others—I've been this way all my life, whether it's giving advice to others on careers, taxes, finances, traveling, or general problem-solving.

Finally, what most qualifies me to help you is that I have successfully used these techniques in my own life.

What have I done? Academically I earned undergraduate degrees in both engineering and liberal arts followed by a graduate degree in management science from Cornell University. The first third of my career was in business analysis and management. The second third was in research and public administration, and the final third in college teaching (math, management and personal growth).

I currently help others as an instructor, author, financial consultant, tax counselor, musician, landlord, career counselor and lender, while furthering my own education as a student and world traveler.

My wife and I have been married for over 30 years. Our two children have completed their formal educations and are now pursuing careers with great care and optimism. We are also experiencing the joys of grandparenting.

Let me assure you, I am not some kind of "guru" and I don't have all the answers. But I have seen too much discontent and frustration out there. There is too much pain and suffering. Too many good people with great potential just need some of the knowledge and experience that I now have and want to share with them. On the next page, you will find a Reader's Contract to help set the tone for our journey together. Please give it your serious consideration.

As you can tell, I sincerely want to help you help yourself to a fuller, richer and happier life. I have personally taken the steps in this book to gain control of my life. I have helped others do these things to take control of their lives. LETS GET STARTED!

Kent McArthur

Reader's Contract

I understand that this book is not just meant to be read, it is meant to be used. In order to realize the benefits described, the "user" must follow the steps in the sequence defined. If trouble is encountered with the process, the Life Planning Institute is available to help "coach" the reader over any stumbling blocks.

By purchasing this book and the associated computer diskette, I agree to take each step <u>that applies to me</u>. I will take all Self-Tests to determine what I need to work on. If appropriate, I will

- Take a Personality Test on the computer,
- Create Audio Tapes to listen to,
- Meditate about my life and myself, and
- Fill out Personal Worksheets and Forms.

I understand that using the techniques described in this book have brought happiness, good health, wealth and wisdom to the author and many other people. There is no guarantee, stated or implied, that everyone will experience the same results.

Agreed by _____ Date _____

Introduction

Think about your life. Seriously, think about it. Are you happy with it? If you hesitated at all, try this simple test: Count out on your fingers the number of things you're doing to make your life full, rich, happy. Be honest!

How many fingers did you count? One? Two? None? Well, if you didn't use very many fingers, you may be

- feeling guilty because you're wasting your life, perhaps using only a fraction of your talents and abilities.

- bouncing from one unhappy or unfulfilling experience to another, resulting in frequent frustration and disappointment.

- suffering the pain and agony of seeing others lead happy and successful lives while you struggle along from day to day.

- ruining your chances to lead a truly fulfilling life by allowing some basic fear - or fears - to keep a stranglehold on you.

- fighting stress and/or illness with or without medication as you try to combat depression.

- feeling hopeless as you wander aimlessly through life and feeling helpless to improve your lot.

- feeling generally discontented, restless, confused or even overwhelmed by life.

If you can identify with any of these situations, this book is for you. In the following pages, I will help you create for yourself, step by step, a life in which happiness is uppermost.

There's one big reason your life isn't heading in the direction you want it to go: YOU ARE NOT IN CONTROL. This book is designed to help you get a better grip on your life. How? By pointing your life in the direction <u>you</u> want it to go. As we embark on this journey together, you'll also add a purpose to your life, not just for now, but until you close your eyes for the last time.

There are probably several reasons why you're not guiding your life in the right direction. In this book, you'll pinpoint which common problems are hampering you, and what to do about them.

First, you may not know yourself. If this is true, you are probably restless and confused, unable to define what you really want out of life or what's good for you.

Second, you may not know why you are here. If you don't know why you are here, you may feel dissatisfied or guilty, or you may just be generally disheartened with your lot in life. This book will help you identify what purpose life holds for you.

Thirdly, maybe you're scared. If so, well, most of us are afraid of something. But fear can stalk your path like a thug in the shadows, robbing you of the opportunity to control your own future. Being afraid can fill your mind with worry, sadness and negative thoughts. This book will help you loosen fear's grip.

Perhaps your life is out-of-balance causing you to have trouble controlling your own destiny. Feelings of being disabled in some way or being powerless have crept into your life. This occurs when you fail to keep your body, mind, emotions and instincts all limber. If you have allowed one or more of these natural gifts to atrophy, YOU ARE NOT IN CONTROL. This book will show you how to detect and then correct any unhealthful imbalances in your life.

Fifth, a too complex life is a life out-of-control. If you are spending too much of your time feeling stressed-out, overwhelmed, or humiliated because you can't keep your promises, it's very difficult to keep your life on track. Complexities are obstacles which need to be overcome before you can sit in the driver's seat. In the pages that follow, you will discover how to simplify your life while maintaining a healthful balance.

If you feel as though you are floundering, sometimes even worthless, you may not have taken the time or exerted the effort to organize your thoughts and give your life purpose. Clear direction is paramount to a life that is going where you want it to go. This book will help you steer your life in the best direction for you--personally.

Another possible reason for not having control is letting your perspective on one of the important aspects of life (career, relationships, spirituality, money) become blurry. Trying to tolerate an incompatible situation can result in guilt, disillusionment, burnout or even chronic disease. An entire chapter will help you zero in on the best ways to deal with these important issues.

Finally, if you don't know the techniques for success used by both businesses and individuals, you will find yourself in a bog of frustration and procrastination. You must get moving on a plan of action in order to start easing the pain in your life. You can make your day-to-day existence feel as good, as rich, as happy, as you want it to be. By the time you finish this book, you will have a plan that's custom-tailored to work for you. Just follow the step-by-step process that has worked for many others.

You've just learned the major steps to happiness, good health, wealth and wisdom. You've just learned how to take control of your life.

● Know yourself (who you are and why you are here)

● Remove the obstacles (fears, imbalances and complexities)

● Make a plan and act on it (organize, review perspective and schedule).

Follow these steps and your life will have a lot less pain and a lot more happiness than you ever imagined.

How many people do you know who are truly happy? Can you honestly say that you wouldn't trade your life for that of anyone else because you find the way your life is going to be so rich, so full of satisfaction and possibilities, that there's hardly room to make it better?

People can be unhappy in many different ways, but you don't have to count them. Just look around and you'll find a lot of people in some degree of pain. For example,

- Too many people live from paycheck to paycheck. Even people who earn thousands of dollars a month are often scrambling to find the money to pay the mortgage, buy the groceries or pay the electric bill. The fear of being one paycheck away from eviction, of being unable to pay for an emergency operation, or of not being able to repair your car can eat into the way you live. This gnawing fear can even make you ill, emotionally and physically. It's like standing next to a cliff in constant panic that someone is about to push you over the edge.

- Half of all marriages in America collapse into divorce. If you're in an unhappy marriage, you may have a wrecking ball for a constant companion. Every part of your life, your emotional well-being, your finances, your job, can be shattered by an unhappy marriage. Your children's happiness can be ruined as well.

- Millions of working people hate their jobs, fear their bosses, and cringe every day at the very real prospect that they could be the next person to be thrown out the door in a fit of corporate downsizing. You spend at least a third of your day at work. With the pressures that downsizing creates, many people are spending ten or twelve hours per day, even more, at work. To be battling inside yourself for so many hours every working day means frustration, ill health and perhaps even thoughts of divorce or suicide.

Ask yourself this question: "Am I happy?" If so, I am pleased for you, pleased that your life is so full. Now ask yourself another question: "Am I healthy, wealthy and wise?" If so, I am truly happy for you. If you answered both these questions with a ringing "yes," then take the book back. You don't need it. But if you hesitated, if you wavered because something inside you said that something is not right with your life, then read on. Together, you and I can do a lot for your life. It's easy, if you just follow the guidelines.

Are you looking for a quick fix? A miracle cure that will turn your life around overnight? This is the WRONG BOOK! If you're willing to settle for long-lasting improvements so that your life becomes closer to your ideal as each year passes, then read on. But be ready to put forth some effort. I can show you the process but only you can tailor the process to meet your individual personality and circumstances.

In particular, you need to make a commitment that you are prepared, with my help, to do the following things.

1) KNOW YOURSELF

You already know this can be a problem, but now take a closer look. Too many people try to become the kind of person their parents, peers or bosses want them to be.

If you're living a life where you're fighting with yourself all the time because you're trying to be somebody you're not, you're heading for trouble. Not just trouble in general. If the way you're living is at war with who you are, you could end up with a lot of physical and emotional problems. You aren't built to withstand the suffering you inflict on yourself for living life in ways that you resent, distrust, or simply don't like.

You need to understand what you can and cannot do. Don't try to be who you are not.

2) MAKE CHANGES

I know, change is unsettling, and most people would rather not disturb the predictability of their existence. One of the most obvious ways to avoid change is to keep repeating old patterns. Repetition may be comforting, but it creates its own problems.

The more caught up you are in a particular way of living, the more making changes becomes like trying to lift a huge block of granite. The longer you wait, the heavier the granite becomes. You may even feel helpless to make changes, and you may even be afraid to change.

If that's your problem, you won't like the results: You will tolerate and rationalize your unhappiness. You'll live a life you don't like until you're planted in the ground or your ashes are tossed into the sea. That's no way to live. Planned change is a sure road to happiness. Besides, change is usually unavoidable. This book is going to show you how to make constructive, positive changes in your life that will bring you lasting happiness.

3) SIMPLIFY

For most people life is complicated and change is happening at an ever-accelerating pace--even if you don't want it to. But even if you are willing to change, just trying to keep up with all the transformations in your own world and the world at large can drain your batteries.

If your reaction to change is to take on too much responsibility and try to control too much, you're heading for pain and suffering. You must learn how to simplify your life to its most important parts and keep it in balance. Simplicity is a virtue.

4) PLAN

Businesses have to know how to plan their future or they will collapse. The same is true for you. You can take control of your life if you plan to simplify it and make it more meaningful. If you don't, you will squander your resources, drift from relationship to relationship and wander aimlessly through your working life.

There are more risks. The results of passively letting circumstances dictate your life are spiritual bankruptcy, constant fantasizing about lost opportunities, and hours and hours spent moaning about how unhappy you are. Nobody wants to listen to or be around that kind of person. And if that person is you, you'll even get tired of listening to your own whining.

You don't have to cringe in a corner wondering what happened to your life. You can change all that. This book will show you how.

What to expect from this book

Consider this book a diagnostic and repair kit. Through this book, you will find out what the problems are in your life and what is undercutting your chances of being happy. Then you will see, step by step, how to fix the problems. You're going to find some surprises. Your pain is not being caused by the usual culprits. It's not your mother, your father, your spouse, your friends, your boss or your government. Look in the mirror: It's YOU.

This book is based on the three-step path to help you live a happier, healthier, wealthier and wiser life:

I   Understanding yourself,

II   Removing the obstacles from your life, and

III   Taking control of your life.

Chapter 1 will help you understand yourself and guide you to the right parts of the book where you can get help for your particular problems. You will diagnose what is causing your feelings of discontent and unhappiness. You will examine your life to see if you are suffering from:

● Not knowing who you really are.

● Being afraid to act on your convictions.

● Living a life that is too complicated or unbalanced.

● Not knowing how to take control of your own future.

Part 1 (Chapters 2 & 3) will help you probe more deeply into your "inner self" and help you find your "place" in life. When you have finished this part, you will better understand who you are, why you are here, and how you are different from everybody else on the planet.

All of this may sound a little mystical, but it's not. The person that is you is the result of a unique recipe. First, blend your genes, upbringing and education. Then stir in what you have experienced socially, culturally, physically, mentally and spiritually. The product of this recipe will be the traits, principles and beliefs that define your personality.

That product is unique: Nobody else walking this earth has your exact genes and experience, and nobody else has your exact traits, principles and beliefs. Nobody--unless you have an identical twin! Chapter 2 will help you to see for yourself just what your individual personality strengths and weaknesses are. Chapters 3 will help you spell out exactly why you are here. This self-knowledge will generate feelings of comfort and self-confidence.

Armed with this new knowledge of your personality and your missions in life, Chapter 4 shows you how to find and confront the fears that get in the way of your taking control of your own destiny. Many people prefer to settle into the Valley of the Familiar instead of plunging into the Jungle of Change. One is settled and comfortable, the other filled with the unknown.

To avoid the unknown, to settle into the familiar, is to wallow in the comfortable while denying your passions, the parts of life that are truly important to you. Once you overcome your fears you will feel energized and free to follow your passions.

Before you plunge into the Jungle, however, you also must remove any other obstacles that are blocking your path. In part, that means insuring that you live a simple life, one that is free of the clutter which can complicate your existence. To be nimble enough to create your own future, you must get rid of any excess baggage. It just weighs you down, keeping your life unbalanced. Chapters 5 and 6 will show you how you can live a fulfilling life by staying in balance and keeping things simple. These are standards by which you will be making the decisions about how you want to live. Upon the completion of these steps you will feel nurtured and unencumbered while enjoying a new-found inner peace.

At this point, you will be ready to map out the direction you want your life to take. Part 3 will show you step by step how to map out your path by creating your own plan for your future. Once you have fashioned this plan, you won't be confused, you won't make decisions reluctantly. You will have created your personal road map to happiness and success.

Reaching this point will be the critical juncture of your life. You will have begun taking control of your life by ripping out the roots of the pain your old way of living have been causing you. At this point, you will start constructing your own road to a happier, healthier, wealthier and wiser life, full of possibilities and promise. You will begin experiencing the joy of living each day to its fullest.

In Part 3 you will also learn a realistic perspective on many of the problems which bleed the fun and the energy out of your life. Many of these problems have kept you from being at the full strength needed to create your own future. The Sections of Chapter 8 will show you how to deal with specific problems, the leeches which can drain the passion from your existence.

If you have difficulty with relationships, there is a Section that will help to guide your thinking and show you the kind of people who best fit with your personality. With your new understanding of whom you are and what your mission in life is, you can find and develop casual and intimate relationships which work. No longer will you stumble from relationship to relationship, feeling drained and disillusioned. Now you can encourage the people who are right for you and develop full, rich relationships which will provide you with great happiness and stability.

If money troubles plague you, there is a Section that will help you put finances into perspective. Money, or the lack of it, doesn't have to burden your life. You will learn the underlying cause of most financial woes and how to make sure you will always have enough to pay for the future you choose to live.

Fear and guilt sit on the shoulders of many people, but you don't have to live with them. The Section on spirituality will spell out for you how to become comfortable with your beliefs and values. Spirituality should bring comfort and peace of mind to your life, instead of burdening it with fear and guilt.

If your job is a source of frustration and dissatisfaction, there is a Section on identifying the "right job" for you. Many people see themselves as only what their job is, and that nothing they are outside work has much value. When you hear people say, "I am an executive," or "I am a teacher," they may actually believe that's <u>all</u> they are. This Section will help you understand the best career for you so that your job brings you enjoyment and success.

Work can also be a source of constant conflict and anxiety, especially in these days of perpetual downsizing. The Section on this occupational hazard will show you how to recognize the symptoms of burnout. It also provides you with a perspective that can make your work both energizing and invigorating.

Another major influence in your life which you cannot control but often have a choice about, regards the weather. Climate can deeply affect your health wherever you live, or wherever you might be moving. You know that having jobs and relationships which are incompatible with your mental and emotional well-being can be stressful and can damage your health. Well, living somewhere that's hard on your physical health can be damaging, too.

This Section will increase your awareness of the importance of climatic conditions when you're considering where you want to move. You may be surprised to know that there is evolving scientific evidence which says that climate can have a profound effect on your health. Science shows that you may be very different from your neighbor in how well you are able to adapt to the climate in which you live.

In the final Chapter of the book I will show you how to put all your goals, plans and perspective into action. By using the same techniques that successful people and businesses have been using for years, you too, will take control of your life. No longer will your thoughts be scattered and your actions put off until tomorrow. By prioritizing your plans, scheduling your actions and monitoring your progress, you will be living the joyful and fulfilling life that you want.

Along the way, you will be encouraged to record your thoughts and ideas on various documents in the book. Please feel free to use these pages as you would a workbook. Some of the forms that you will create are so important to the overall process of Taking Control of Your Life that I have designated them as "KEEPERS." They are reproduced in a separate Forms Section. They are all in one place so that you can easily find them whenever you need to refer to them during any step in the process. The pages containing the "KEEPERS" have been perforated so that you can remove them from the book for easy duplication. Even if the results of your diagnostic efforts indicate that you can skip a chapter, please complete the "KEEPER" for that chapter. You will need that personal information during a subsequent step.

Finally, if you want to dive into any subject of this book more deeply, the Annotated Bibliography will provide you with an ocean of references. It also includes a helpful review of the importance and approach for every book listed. The entries are categorized and cross-referenced to all of the major segments of the book, including: Philosophy of Life, Simplicity, Understanding Yourself, Goal Setting, Life Planning, Spirituality, Finances, Career Planning and more.

How to use this book

Don't expect to become happy, healthy, wealthy and wise within 36 hours after skimming through this book for the first time. Nothing which offers truly lasting benefits comes that easily. This book is meant to be a very personal experience between you (someone who sincerely wants to be happy) and me, your coach (who also wants you to be happy).

To start troubleshooting your life, I have included several diagnostic kits to help you understand who you are and what the sources of your unhappiness are. Just reading about these tools won't make them work. You have to use them. That means taking some simple tests, sometimes grading and interpreting them, and always understanding the results in order to raise your level of awareness.

This book doesn't stop at diagnosing your problems. Instead you will find several techniques for improving your life. Again, just reading about how to make improvements may be entertaining, but it won't bring you any closer to controlling your life and building a happiness-filled future. You need to put these tools to work. You have to use the tools and apply them in the ways that I show you if you expect to get the benefits.

Don't expect to complete the process you will find here in one sitting. Or two. Or three. Or even a week. You'll find much to absorb and to think about here, and some new ways of looking at and doing things that you will have to become used to. But, each step is designed to be very doable and bring you immediate results.

As you work your way through the process, remember, we're talking about the entire rest of your life here. So, make the commitment. Take the time your life deserves and use this book properly. You deserve the attention. You deserve the fun. You deserve the happiness.

Chapter 1

Diagnostic SELF-TESTS:
Pointing You in the Right Direction

Here you're going to help yourself "zero in" on how to go about using this book. You don't want to waste your time and energy on problems you don't have. You need to focus on the chapters that will give you help where you need it.

This chapter is a kind of diagnostic kit. It will help you look closely at the four major reasons for unhappiness. You'll look at them one by one. Then you'll decide for yourself whether you have to grapple with one or more of these problems to increase your chances of being happy, healthy, wealthy and wise.

You'll also begin to learn some skills basic to improving your life. These steps—the Getting Ready steps—are

- Knowing yourself and why you are here.

- Overcoming your fears and excuses for not taking action.

- Simplifying and balancing your life.

But more about these steps later.

You may think that being happy, healthy, wealthy and wise sounds like a fantasy. Well, it isn't. Happiness is not an altered state of consciousness. You don't have to be hallucinating in order to be happy. Look around you. Surely, you know people who don't worry about having enough money who treasure their relationships with their family.

On the job, you know people who don't undercut or stab co-workers and managers in the back. Instead, they cultivate ways of working together in a team effort to make their company or their organization both productive and enjoyable.

You also know people who push their bodies, their minds and their spirits to make themselves grow and learn so they become filled with the richness of living. They expect health, wealth, wisdom and happiness to come their way. And they get what they expect. Certainly they don't get it all the time, in all ways, but their lives are constantly blossoming and being fulfilled. Know what? You can too.

If you're not at that point, this book will help you help yourself. If you are living your life mostly by putting up with unhappiness and dissatisfaction, you need to change. If you see others having more money than you do; if you see people whose careers are fun and rewarding; if you see people whose moments are mostly filled with a passion for living and ample rewards for doing what they're doing; and you see very little of all that in your own life—well, you know there must be more. You just don't know how to get what you want. This book will point the way.

In this chapter, we will pinpoint the specific problems you need to work on. Later, you'll find a road map showing you how to stop sidetracking yourself. You will create your own path to a life that will make you happy and proud to be who you are.

First things first. And that means answering the questions in this chapter. Although this diagnostic kit is divided into four Self-Tests, you should work your way through all of the questions in one sitting. If you do, you will be honest with yourself and you will achieve the maximum benefit that these exercises have to offer.

You see, they have been empirically calibrated to help you honestly examine your thoughts and feelings so you can spend your time fixing only the problems that you have. You can skip the remedy for problems that, for you, don't exist.

It's almost like going to the doctor. Before the doctor can prescribe a treatment, he or she has to know what your ailment is. You wouldn't want the doctor to prescribe medicine you don't need or treatments which won't fix the problem you have. Well, you don't want to spend your time "fixing" something inside you that isn't broken, either. Ready? Here we go!

> "Every man is the Architect
>
> of his own future."
>
> —Appius Claudius

Self-Test #1

Give yourself a score ranging from 0 to 10 for each question.

NEVER RARELY SOMETIMES OFTEN USUALLY ALWAYS
  0   2   4   6   8   10

1 __2__1. I try new experiences expecting to find enjoyment only to be disappointed.

4 __8__2. I am under a lot of stress.

4 __6__3. I feel as though I'm "going against the tide."

2 __4__4. I doubt my own judgment.

2 __6__5. I am unhappy at work or school.

0 __7__6. I blame others for my dissatisfaction.

2 __6__7. I find it difficult to make decisions.

4 __8__8. I associate with people who sap my energy.

2 __8__9. I feel that my talents are being wasted.

2 __6__10. I run out of energy trying to meet the expectations of others.

2 __4__11. I have trouble communicating with others.

4 __9__12. I am dissatisfied with my home environment.

2 __2__13. I am uncomfortable with the role I play at work.

0 __3__14. Life moves too fast for me.

2 __5__15. I find myself daydreaming, uncertain of what to do next.

0 __6__16. I envy other people who can get things done.

2 __6__17. I take aspirin or other painkilling drugs.

2 __4__18. I find it difficult to get a deep, refreshing sleep.

0 __2__19. I believe that other people's success is due mainly to luck.

0 __2__20. I feel like "a square peg in a round hole."

35 104 TOTAL POINTS
     4

Self-Test #2

Give yourself a score ranging from 0 to 10 for each question.

NEVER RARELY SOMETIMES OFTEN USUALLY ALWAYS
  0   2   4   6   8   10

5 _5_ 1. I gravitate toward activities that are adventuresome.

8 _5_ 2. I like to try new things.

6 _5_ 3. I set goals for myself.

3 _3_ 4. I am able to commit to a relationship to the exclusion of others.

4 _5_ 5. I can concentrate totally on one project until it is completed.

8 _4_ 6. I am secure in my opinions.

10 _5_ 7. I look forward to the changes that the future will bring.

8 _8_ 8. I handle my responsibilities in a timely manner.

6 _4_ 9. I plan ahead.

6 _4_ 10. I enjoy overcoming obstacles.

8 _4_ 11. I like to turn problems into opportunities.

10 _10_ 12. I think it is silly for someone to spend time hoping that their life will work out someday.

10 _10_ 13. I see myself making a difference in the world.

8 _4_ 14. I thoroughly enjoy myself.

6 _5_ 15. I act on my good ideas.

8 _5_ 16. I am confident about my skills and abilities.

10 _7_ 17. I have many good friends.

10 _8_ 18. I do my best when no one is watching.

2 _5_ 19. I think it is stupid for people to act on their superstitions.

6 _2_ 20. I find it difficult to become humiliated by others.

108 TOTAL POINTS

13

Self-Test #3

Give yourself a score ranging from 0 to 10 for each question.

NEVER RARELY SOMETIMES OFTEN USUALLY ALWAYS
   0   2   4   6   8   10

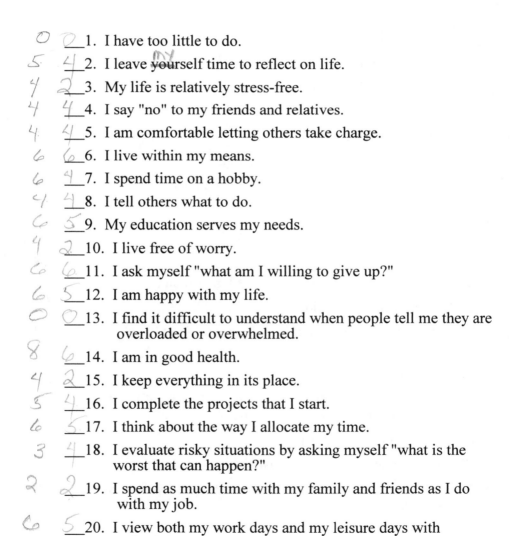

O   *2* 1. I have too little to do.

5   *4* 2. I leave yourself time to reflect on life.

4   *2* 3. My life is relatively stress-free.

4   *4* 4. I say "no" to my friends and relatives.

4   *4* 5. I am comfortable letting others take charge.

6   *6* 6. I live within my means.

6   *4* 7. I spend time on a hobby.

4   *4* 8. I tell others what to do.

6   *5* 9. My education serves my needs.

4   *2* 10. I live free of worry.

6   *6* 11. I ask myself "what am I willing to give up?"

6   *5* 12. I am happy with my life.

O   *O* 13. I find it difficult to understand when people tell me they are overloaded or overwhelmed.

8   *6* 14. I am in good health.

4   *2* 15. I keep everything in its place.

5   *4* 16. I complete the projects that I start.

6   *5* 17. I think about the way I allocate my time.

3   *4* 18. I evaluate risky situations by asking myself "what is the worst that can happen?"

2   *2* 19. I spend as much time with my family and friends as I do with my job.

6   *5* 20. I view both my work days and my leisure days with enthusiasm.

89   *74* TOTAL POINTS

Self-Test #4

Answer True or False to each statement.

N 1. I have a definite purpose in my life.

N 2. I experience relatively little stress.

N 3. I keep my life very simple.

N 4. I "go with the flow" around me.

N 5. I keep my life in balance at all times.

N 6. I know what activities energize me.

N 7. I set long-range goals for myself.

N 8. I establish action plans to structure my life.

N 9. I monitor my progress toward my objectives.

N 10. I talk to myself on a regular basis.

N 11. My life has a sense of meaning to it.

Y 12. I have a philosophy of life.   "I don't know"

N 13. I devote myself to causes that are larger than me.

N 14. I know where I'm going in my life.

N 15. I often ask myself "what is really great in my life right now?"

Y 16. I plan to reach my potential.

N 17. I never feel that things beyond my control are stopping me from achieving what I want in life.

N 18. Things generally go my way.

Y 19. I enjoy contemplating alternatives for my future.

Y 20. I always enjoy accomplishing something for which I've been striving.

4 TOTAL NUMBER OF <u>TRUE</u> RESPONSES

Evaluating and Interpreting Self-Test #1   *105*

The first step toward taking control of your life is understanding yourself. No matter how much education you have, how much money you earn or how many people you know in high places, you will never be happy if you don't know who you are. If you haven't taken the time to properly identify the resources and limitations you have, it is pure luck if you have been putting those resources to good use. Let's see if you know who you really are.

LOW SCORES

35
1/23/13

Surprise! A low score here is something to be proud of. If you scored from 0-66 on Diagnostic #1, you know yourself quite well. You may have come to this point in a variety of ways. Maybe it was self-examination. Maybe it was feedback from personality testing. Maybe it was a combination of those or something else. However you did it, give yourself a huge pat on the back. Your happiness is not crimped by your not knowing who you really are.

That means that Chapters 2 & 3, the ones that include some personality testing, will only be useful if you want to fine-tune your knowledge about yourself. You may learn a few things, but you won't feel your world being rocked by what you see there. You understand a great deal of it already. You will want to spend more time on the areas revealed by any of the next three diagnostic tests in which you may actually need some work.

Let me say congratulations! You have an excellent grasp of who you are and why you are here. You're well on your way to a life of good health, wealth, wisdom and happiness. I suggest you go directly to KEEPER #2—MY MISSION STATEMENTS and write down your missions in life. You will want this information for later steps as you continue to give your life the direction it needs for a future of success and fulfillment.

MEDIUM SCORES 105

If you scored 67-133 points, you know a lot about yourself. But, you also have much to learn. Chapter 2 will be important to you because you need to fully grasp who you are before you can make the important choices in your life. Those choices include relationships, career, religion, education, lifestyle and where it is best for you to live and work. But more about those topics later.

If you don't understand who you are, then you are making these choices blindfolded. Good decisions will probably be the result of pure chance. More likely, you could spend the rest of your life having to adjust to bad choices. Or, you could start over again and again, never enjoying the richness of fulfillment that sound life decisions will bring.

Let me give you an example from my own life: My son bounced around from one occupation to another. And he bounced hard. Taxidermist, drummer in a rock band, recording technician, psychological counselor, he tried them all. Then he took a personality test which showed that he was best suited for something no one, least of all himself, had ever suspected. The test said that my son would make a terrific physical therapist.

He gave this some serious thought. Once he decided to take the plunge and become a physical therapist, big chunks of the rest of his life started to fall into place. He knew what kind of education he wanted. His spiritual perspective took shape. His long-term relationship matured with the woman who would become his wife. And, their lifestyle has flourished along with their bank account. My son is a much happier, healthier, wealthier and wiser person. As a result, he and his wife have made appropriate and confident geographical and family decisions.

HIGH SCORES

If you scored between 134-200, I have bad news. You made it this far in life knowing very little about how you are different from other people. By not knowing who you really are, you haven't been able to define what you're doing on the face of this planet or where you want to go.

You probably have been wandering aimlessly, meandering through your existence, making false starts, doing things for the wrong reasons, experiencing more than your share of frustrations. Maybe you drifted from relationship to relationship rather than making long-term commitments to friendships and intimate relationships that really work. You have most likely experienced very little of the joy and fulfillment life has in store for you.

Your life can be different. When you know who you are and why you are here, what your strengths and weaknesses are, and how they complement other people, your life will be very different. You can commit to healthy and long-lasting relationships. You can find the occupations in life that give you satisfaction, fulfillment and ultimately money. You can become a richer person in many ways. You can do it. This book will show you how.

My cousin fell victim to the problems suffered by people who don't know themselves well. She ended up in a marriage that didn't work. She had two children before she came eyeball to eyeball with how miserable her marriage made her. Fortunately, she took some personality tests and was able to better understand herself and face the nature of her predicament.

As a result, she decided to dive into her longstanding interest in psychology by earning her Master's degree in counseling. Then she took a counseling job at her daughter's school. After much marriage counseling, she and her husband divorced. She also took a very long, hard look at the people she considered friends. She decided that she was compatible with only one. The others disappeared from her life.

The process wasn't as fast as whipping up a batch of instant pudding or opening a car door. It took her five years. But if she hadn't taken the personality tests to rediscover who she really is, she never would have identified the problems or faced them. Once she did, she worked her way into an occupation which she loves, formed relationships which are satisfying, earned the love and respect of her children and made enough money to own her own home. She also is now spiritually grounded in a strong system of family values.

Evaluating and Interpreting Self-Test #2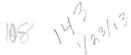

Even after you understand who you are and why you are here, you may have obstacles standing in the way of your happiness. The second major task while getting ready to take control of your life is confronting fears and discarding excuses you may have for not taking action.

You will never fulfill your purpose and enjoy success in life if you allow such obstacles to control your life. Your score on Self-Test #2 will tell you how much work you must do to eliminate any fears and excuses that are standing in the way of the health, wealth, wisdom and happiness you deserve and can have. Let's look.

HIGH SCORES

If you scored in the 134-200 point range, WHOA. Step back and look at yourself in the mirror. You have nerves of steel. You know no fear! Well, at least you don't show any signs of the fears which most commonly paralyze people and keep them from moving ahead in their lives. Even so, you probably will want to scan Chapter 4 to make sure that one of the major fears this part examines doesn't apply to you. Check out Table II—Some Common Fears with Substitute Messages for Your Subconscious beginning on page 142. If none of these fears send shivers up your spine, terrific. If you do find one, you need to confront that fear before moving on to other chapters.

One common fear is a fear of the unknown. People often reveal that they have this fear in subtle ways. The most common one is that they don't want to move far from home. Any thoughts about relocating are squelched almost as soon as they come up. This fear extends far, far beyond just wanting to live with the known, the comfortable, the predictable, the familiar, and nothing else. It is a genuine mistrust of the unknown—perhaps even terror.

For example, a number of people I know from my tiny home town are still living there after many, many years. Often they haven't budged more than a few blocks from where they grew up. Even if they have moved across town, they're not willing to move out of it.

I saw this fear most clearly when I returned for my high school's 25th reunion and ran into the boy who had been my idol on the baseball team. Everyone had thought he'd get a baseball scholarship and maybe even make the big leagues. But he was afraid to leave home. He was still there 25 years later, tending bar.

Curious about why he remained there, I decided to ask him. He told me how little he liked his life there, how he always needed more money, that he didn't do much and didn't want to. It was clear to me after 15 minutes of conversation that he didn't like his life in our hometown, but he was too scared of what was beyond its borders to ever leave.

MEDIUM SCORES 108

A score in the 67-133 range says: though you have generally guided your life along a satisfying and fulfilling path, minor obstacles are cluttering it. Being afraid is a marginal problem for you. It's essential to have the smallest number of fears and hangups as possible weighing you down as you walk along the path that will take you toward a life full of promise. So, plan on spending some time with Chapter 4, which will help you put any of the major fears into perspective. Then you can remove them without shame, embarrassment or hesitation.

A client of mine serves as an excellent example of people who can know themselves well, but just can't pull their lives together. In fact, "Sam" knows himself very well. He knows he has a strong entrepreneurial streak and that his personality matches well with four or five career possibilities.

Sam could start a terrific business in many diverse areas. He could be a financial planner or a personnel manager. He also excels at travel coordinating, personal coaching, communications consulting and—would you believe it?—general contracting.

The problem: Sam is afraid of failure. He has so much interest in each of those fields that he can't—or won't—make a choice. He says he's afraid he won't be able to do justice to his other interests. Instead of going full throttle for a career that he knows would suit him well, he fritters his life away working the counter at a car rental agency. There he reads, studies and fantasizes about starting businesses in all of the areas where he could excel. He has a safe fantasy life, but his working life is boring and dissatisfying and hardly pays the bills.

His problem is a common one for people making their first career choice. They're often worried about committing themselves to making a career decision which means spending more time in one of their areas of interest, while necessarily spending less time in others.

This client of mine is, of course, an extreme example. When it comes to making a career choice, he is frozen in his tracks. Because he's scared to death that he will fail, he doesn't try to accomplish anything. That way he can't fail or suffer the humiliation that goes with failure.

Instead of living his own life, he lives everyone else's. He helps friends, neighbors, relatives achieve their goals and objectives. He can experience the thrill of their victories while not risking his own defeat.

Sam doesn't realize that if he would get past his fear of failure and humiliation, he could create his own identity and live a more satisfying life. If you have tendencies in this direction, Chapter 4 will show you how to beat your fear of failure or your fear of change or whatever fear you may be harboring.

LOW SCORES

A score of 0-66 shows that you have some latent fears which need to be addressed before you can get on with the process of becoming a happy person. Chapter 4 will help you work your way through some of the most common problems on a step-by-step basis.

The fear of change is probably the most basic and most prevalent of these. I have encountered it frequently among career planning clients I have counseled.

A typical scenario is for people to go through the entire counseling program with great enthusiasm. Then they balk when the results suggest that they should make a career change. Obviously, they came to me hoping that I would confirm the wisdom of their current career choice because they were afraid to make a change.

This fear is sometimes so consuming that not even the results of counseling dissuades them. Even when my counseling clearly shows that their current career requires them to play a role which is incompatible with their personality (causing them tremendous job stress that carries over into their personal life), they are reluctant to change. Chapter 4 provides the real guidance that these people need: How to overcome the fear of change.

A variation of this problem is the fear of failure. I have another client who refuses to establish goals because she feels she would just be setting herself up for failure. Her attitude is: Why should I risk trying to achieve anything? If I fail, I will just suffer tremendous humiliation.

She prefers instead to support others in their endeavors. By helping friends, neighbors and relatives achieve their goals and objectives, she can share in the "thrill of victory" without feeling responsible for the "agony of defeat." However, this approach frequently results in her getting stressed out because the others "take her for granted" or "expect too much of her" or "just use her."

What she doesn't realize is if she would overcome her fear of failure (and the implied humiliation) she could do a lot for herself. She could establish her own identity, raise her level of self-esteem and relate to others on a stress-free, collaborative basis which would result in everyone around her being happier. If you have tendencies in this direction, Chapter 4 will show you how to combat this phobia and the related fear of change.

Evaluating and Interpreting Self-Test #3

Your prospect for happiness increases dramatically when you lead a balanced life. That's when you exercise all of your faculties: body, mind, emotions, and intuition. If you are out of balance, your "parts" will not be in sync. Some will suffer overuse while others are allowed to atrophy. This condition is not healthy and can be a major source of frustration and dissatisfaction in your life.

You've also got to have room in your life for the changes you're going to make. That means you must simplify your life by eliminating any clutter that may have accumulated. Clutter consists of the parts of your life that stand in the way of your getting where you want to go. This debris can sidetrack you from the path you want to follow. You will end up wasting your time doing things that distract you from what you should be doing.

The result of simplifying your life is that you give yourself breathing room. It's like having unwelcome guests staying in your home. They never seem to leave and you can't get them to leave, no matter how much you want them to go. Simplifying your life is how you usher out your life's unwelcome guests and start to live your own life again.

The results of Self-Test #3 will show you whether your life is balanced and whether it is simple enough to accommodate change. If it isn't, then you will have to lean heavily on Chapters 5 and 6. These two chapters will show you how to eliminate clutter, restore balance, and give yourself the time and energy you need to make the improvements that will turn your life around.

HIGH SCORES

If you scored between 134-200, you have managed to keep your life relatively simple and in good balance. You are not burdened with demands that waste your time and energy. You are devoting ample time to all areas of your life. Scanning Chapters 5 and 6 briefly will probably be all you'll need.

When you do scan, you may run across an idea or two which will help you in simplifying your life further. Such changes could bring you huge rewards by freeing up the time you need to give your life new direction and improve the overall quality of your life.

For example, I cut my own grass for years until I reached the point where I despised doing it. I kept telling myself that doing the grass was giving me some good exercise and saved the cost of having someone else do it.

Then one summer my wife and I were going to take an extended vacation. I was forced to look around for a gardener to take care of things while we were gone. When we returned, the lawn was a rich green and the envy of the neighborhood. The price was so reasonable I hired the gardener on a permanent basis.

What a relief! I had lifted the burden of a chore that I hated from my shoulders. I put it on somebody who knew how to do it well. Instead of begrudgingly pushing a roaring machine back and forth while my body was sweating and stinking, I spent that time walking or riding a bike with my wife. I feel foolish for not having made this simplification and re-balancing a long time ago. What a real quality-of-life improvement.

You probably have several quality-of-life improvements you can make in your life. Before going through Chapter 6, look at KEEPER #5—MY WHEEL OF BALANCE. Think about ways you can simplify your life by substituting a fulfilling activity for something that you hate doing. Take note of these potential changes. You'll be glad you did! It will help you get ready to begin taking control of your life.

MEDIUM SCORES 74   83

Scoring 67-133 means you can improve the quality of your life by creating a better balance, simplifying your existence, or both. Chapters 5 and 6 will help you considerably. They will show you step-by-step how to go about bringing balance into your life while you're ushering complexity out.

Think about it: One of the biggest resources every one of us has is TIME. Whether we're rich or poor, we all have the same amount at our disposal every day. However, you "spend" your time differently than everyone else. It's one way you are different from all other people on earth.

Nobody uses his or her time quite the same way as you use yours. There are so many different areas of life in which you can spend your time: family and friends, career, finances, health, spirituality, education, and hobbies just to name a few. The fulfillment you experience in your life depends to some extent on the balance you achieve among these competing demands on your time.

It's difficult to read about a philosophy of life without encountering balance as an essential ingredient in the search for happiness. But that philosophy is not just found in books. You yourself know people who seem to have a handle on their lives, who are quite busy but still seem to have time for the important things.

You don't have to watch them. You can be one of them. But if you neglect one or more of the major areas of your life, the overall quality of your life will suffer. You know plenty of people who are so caught up in doing one thing, such as work, that the other areas of their lives shrivel up for lack of attention. Don't let that happen to you. And if it already has happened, then stop hurting yourself like that.

A few years ago, I had a boss in the business world who held a very high corporate job which suited his personality well. "Jim" had a college degree, he was married, and he earned a generous salary. He had what many people would consider a full and perhaps even an ideal life.

Not true. Jim let his job rule his life. He was out of the house very early in the morning and sometimes didn't get home until midnight. His life was out of balance. He was soon working on his second marriage. Jim's second wife had the same complaint as the first: He treated her as impersonally and dictatorially as he treated any of his employees. The people he called his friends actually were workplace acquaintances, people with whom he spent many hours but didn't know very well at all.

Even his money was a source of grief. Jim was making so much of it he was constantly looking for places in which to invest. The trouble was, he didn't take the time to research his investments. Instead, he just put money down on his hunches or tips from people he knew or followed a stock broker's suggestions. He lost a lot of money that way, and he couldn't understand why. His life was completely out of balance.

A few years after I left the company, Jim had burned himself out. The strategies, the clear thinking, the energy, the passion he'd had for his work, had all been spent. He had nothing in his life to replace his obsession with work. But the company considered him to be replaceable, and he was pushed out in the street. His unbalanced life had caught up with him, and he paid a very heavy price.

Don't be like my former boss. If you are spending too much time in one area of your life and neglecting the others, Chapters 5 and 6 will show you how to get back on track. Remember, your life must be balanced and simple before you can begin traveling that road toward fulfillment.

LOW SCORES

If your score for Self-Test #3 was in the 0-66 range, your life is too complex for your own good. You need to take out your machete and hack away at the cluttered tangle your life has become. Chapter 6 will show you how to cut away the deadwood and start to stimulate your own growth by giving your life room to breathe.

Incidentally, simplifying your life also gives you an opportunity to organize it. When your life is organized, you can do more without becoming confused and upset when you can't find the information (or person or item) that you're looking for. If you don't have a system for running your life, you risk having all that complexity creep back in without your even noticing.

I have another client who is constantly unorganized. "Ben" is adventuresome. He knows his own strengths and weaknesses, but he keeps butting up against his own disorganization whenever he tries to accomplish anything that will bring him happiness.

Ben's enthusiasm for new projects is like a rocket blasting off the launch pad. But, soon his interest fizzles and he moves on to a new project. When he returns to a prior project, he can't remember where things are, so he has to start over. What a waste! He's always hunting around his office or house for something that he's lost.

This man was a highly successful entrepreneur when he had a personal assistant to track and administer these details. Now that he doesn't have an assistant he's constantly frustrated by his own personal disorganization. The result: He wastes unnecessary amounts of time and money without making very much progress toward his goals in life.

Does this problem sound familiar? If you suffer from clutter, imbalance and disorganization, Chapter 6 will show you how to simplify, create the balance, and fashion the organization you need to prepare you for taking control of your life and making it far more satisfying than it is today.

Evaluating and Interpreting Self-Test #4

Even if you did well on the first three self-tests, that doesn't mean you've got your life where you want it. You could still be wandering aimlessly, wondering why you are not happier, why you don't have a better grip on your life and why you're not satisfied with the way things are going for you. You still have something gnawing at your brain that tells you life just isn't giving you what you want.

There's probably a good reason. You see, the first three steps are really just stages of getting ready. The fourth step is where you stop getting ready to do something with your life. Here is where you take action. Here is where you start doing it. In this stage, you stop getting ready and you start aiming your life in the direction that will bring you fulfillment and success.

Aim? Yes. It is here where you define where you want your life to go. This is where you map out the journey you want to take and where you want it to lead. It's always easier to get somewhere if you know where you want to go. And that's what this stage is all about. The results of Self-Test #4 will tell you the extent to which you already have begun to create your own road map by giving your life direction.

HIGH SCORES

If you got a 15 or higher, well, congratulations. You're already practicing many of the successful planning techniques which have brought many other people happiness, good health, wealth and wisdom. In fact, I'd really like to hear from you so I can chronicle your success and others can learn from what you've done.

However, if you're still

- not living the kind of life you want,

- feeling that your life is a little hollow,

- thinking that something constantly is getting in the way of your happiness,

then odds are that you have some work to do in the Getting Ready Steps. You remember those:

- Knowing yourself and why you are here.

- Overcoming your fears and excuses for not taking action.

- Simplifying and balancing your life.

So, although your score says you can just skim Part 3, consider reviewing it in some detail once you have completed your preparation for taking control of your life. It is very probable that your current goals and plans will not produce the happiness you deserve if they are not based on the new you.

Who is that? That's the You who understands who you are, is free of crippling fears and excuses, and leads a simple but balanced life. Anyway, be sure to fill out KEEPER #8—MY LONG-TERM SCHEDULE. If you have a good grasp of the planning techniques explained in Part 3, this Keeper will enable you to achieve direction and control of your future.

MEDIUM SCORES

A score in the 8-14 range suggests that you have taken partial control of your life. However, your ability to direct your life toward the future that you want still leaves some room for improvement.

Chapter 7 will help you get yourself pointed in the right direction. It will help you fill in the missing pieces so you can take control of your own destiny. You need to use the tools that business people have been using for years to ensure that their organizations will endure. These are the techniques you will learn in this chapter so you can corner your share of happiness.

These techniques aren't taught in school, though they ought to be. They are not part of any organized religion. They don't appear as the answers on any television game shows. However, every successful businessperson knows how well these techniques work to make organizations robust and productive.

Guess what? They work the same way for real people. Applying these tools can make your life robust, productive, and fulfilling. Don't waste any more time wandering around looking for some direction in your life. It's useless to hope that someone will magically tell you what you want and how to go about getting it. Magic wands and genies belong in cartoons. For real life, turn to Chapter 7 and begin to create your own path toward the destination you want.

LOW SCORES

A score in this self-test of seven or less means that this book, and Part 3 in particular, could be one of the most important experiences of your life. I don't say that just to make you feel good that you bought this book or to make myself look important. I know these techniques work because I've used them, and so have many people I have worked with.

These step-by-step techniques have let me make changes in my life while enjoying the kind of happiness, health, wealth and wisdom that I want to have. Sure, like anything worthwhile, it takes some time and some discipline, but each step of the way is quite easy.

When you start using these tools, you can begin your journey in the direction you want to travel. This is how you will take charge of your life and transform your feelings of helplessness and despair into feelings of fulfillment and satisfaction.

OK, now you know where you stand. You know what you need to work on and what you already do pretty well. To recap,

- If you've been lax in understanding yourself and your purpose in life, head straight for Part 1.

- If you're harboring some fears and hiding behind some excuses that you need to root out, spend time with Chapter 4.

- If your life is cluttered with complexities or out of balance, the step-by-step procedures in Chapters 5 and 6 will clear away what is not essential and help you get re-balanced.

- If you need to learn how to fashion a plan for your life that will work for you, then Part 3 holds the key.

But REMEMBER, as straightforward as each of these steps may be, this is a <u>sequential process</u>. You must do it in order if you want to achieve the desired results. First, you need to understand yourself and your mission or else you can't face your fears. If you don't face your fears, you can't distinguish those aspects of your life which keep you from getting where you want to go. By conquering your fears you will free up the energy that your fears have been consuming. Then you will be able to make changes that are in your own best interest.

Only then can you actually simplify your life, clearing away the clutter of unnecessary activities and the de-energizing forces in your life. You must clear away whatever bleeds your spirit of the time and energy you need so you can create and put into motion your plan for your own future. That future is the one you want. It's time to discard the life you have bitterly accepted. Now you know how to make yourself happy.

Sound complicated? Sound difficult? Believe me, it isn't. It's as natural as the passing of the four seasons. *You just have to start doing it step by step.* You'll always find that you are ready for the next step just as the one you're completing is coming to its logical end.

> "The future is not something we enter. The future is something we create."
> —Leonard I. Sweet

Part 1

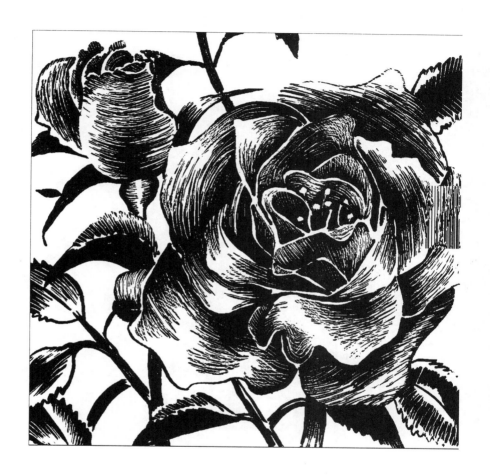

Understanding
Yourself

Chapter 2

How to Determine Who You Are

The most important step you can take toward being happy is understanding yourself. If you can't recognize who you are, you won't know what really makes you happy or unhappy. In this chapter you will discover or rediscover this special resource, *you* by

- taking a personality test to identify the *real you*,

- reviewing the meaning of such things as traits, roles, beliefs, and principles,

- imagining your own eulogy that identifies the *ideal you*, and

- summarizing your personality highlights on KEEPER #1—MY RESOURCES.

Taking these steps will bring you the self-confidence and peace of mind you need to take control of your life.

Because of its importance, you will also find KEEPER #1—MY RESOURCES in the KEEPER Forms Section for easy reference. That section contains all of the research you will be doing on yourself as you map out the journey that represents the rest of your life. Being in one location, they will be easy to find when you need to use them. Since these pages are perforated, they can also be removed easily for copying.

MY RESOURCES is your summary of your personality. This information will form the foundation of your thinking as you begin to take control of your life. It needs to be accurate because it is the building block upon which everything else depends.

You most likely have several misconceptions about yourself which can distort how you look at yourself and who you believe you are. These distortions are like a fun house mirror: you see an image that somewhat resembles you, but it's not a true reflection. MY RESOURCES is meant to give you a true mirror of who you are.

> "It's not what we don't know that hurts. It's what we know that ain't so."   —Will Rogers

How you define what it means to be happy, healthy, wealthy and wise is as individual as the clothes you wear. Like clothing, when it comes to happiness, there's no such thing as "one size fits all." The only way to know what suits you, what fits you personally, is to understand *you*. If you don't understand yourself, you cannot be happy. It's as simple as that.

Why? Because to be happy, you have to know who you are and what will make you happy. The path you decide to take toward that happiness will be the path that is best for you and you alone. If you want to be happy, healthy, wealthy and wise, you first have to be yourself. This chapter is designed to help you figure out just who it is that you are. You are the "resource" you have to work with as you begin to take control of your life.

Don't think of this book as you would a cheap novel you can buy at any drugstore. It's not designed to be used once, then discarded. It's meant to be a long-lasting reference, something you can turn to again when you have the need to make important life choices. Consider it a lifelong companion, not a quick fix.

Look. You can't pin your hopes for happiness on other people. Not your parents, brothers, sisters, friends, teachers or bosses. You can't imitate someone you admire. Trying to be like someone else is like trying to put on their clothing. It will never fit you in appearance, style or fashion, the way your own clothes do. You have chosen your wardrobe to suit your personal and particular taste. The path you take toward happiness, good health, wealth and wisdom should be selected the same way.

There is great danger in trying to be a carbon copy of someone else. Trying to be someone else means following <u>their</u> path, not yours. That path will only lead to disappointment, frustration, stress, failure, ill health and a sense that your life isn't really your own. Which, of course, it won't be.

Thinking and acting like the person you are—*that's you, and nobody else*—is the only way to take charge of the life that is yours. It is the only way to create the future that fits you.

Of course, there may be other reasons you haven't taken the time to figure out who you are. You may have been a passive person, just watching the world go by, instead of trying to interact in your own best interests. Now you've decided it's time to take action, to grip your life hard and turn it in the direction you want it to go.

Then again, maybe you're going through a big change in your life: a divorce, a family death, the loss of a job, or a long illness. Maybe it's a desire to just do something different with your life. Whatever your reason for deciding to whip your life into shape, it's a goal well worth achieving. This book was written for you.

You must understand who you are so that you can make choices that will make your life fulfilling. Knowing who you are allows you to find roles in life which are comfortable. This means you need to understand and **be** yourself in order to choose:

- A career which is compatible with who you are, where you will find fulfillment while contributing, directly or indirectly, to the lives of others.

- A compatible mate with whom you can build a strong emotional life together.

- A compatible lifestyle in which you can experience peace and inner harmony.

- A level and breadth of formal and informal education which will satisfy your intellectual curiosity.

- A place to live which is both compatible with who you are and will provide you a healthful physical environment.

You can achieve all five of these ingredients of a happy and fulfilling life only if you first take the time to understand yourself. YOUR MAJOR LIFE DECISIONS MUST BE BASED ON WHO YOU REALLY ARE, NOT WHAT WORKS FOR SOMEONE ELSE.

Let me give you two examples—one famous, one personal—of people who made their lives miserable because they didn't pay attention to who they are. Jay Leno is a good illustration of what happens to a person who tries to be someone he isn't.

A few years ago, Leno took over NBC's Tonight Show and immediately started copying the format of his mentor, Johnny Carson. But, what had worked so well for Johnny failed miserably for Jay. The show's ratings nosedived. The program was being panned nearly every day by the critics, and the competition's ratings were so much better it was embarrassing.

Then Leno decided to be himself. He decided to draw on his own experiences and temperament; he decided to use his own style, not that of someone else. Jay made the show an expression of his own personality. Guess what? The audience came back, and Leno's show became the most highly rated in that time slot, just because he decided to be himself.

It's not just the rich and famous who can tumble into the trap of imitation, of trying to be like people they're not. We all fall into it from time to time. You have probably tried to imitate others because you liked and respected them. My own cousin suffered when she made this mistake. She tried to be like her mother: a terrific wife, parent and homemaker.

Well, her mother's temperament was completely compatible with her caregiver role. She thoroughly enjoyed the years when her children were growing up. In fact, she enjoyed the caregiver role so much that after raising them, she found others to care for. She spent ten years living with and caring for three relatives who needed her help.

But that wasn't the kind of person my cousin was. My cousin was not interested in caregiving. From her earliest days, she loved to read books, argue about every topic imaginable or work with a friend on some deep intellectual problem. Cooking a meal, driving an ungrateful child to a baseball game or dance class, well, those activities were not her idea of fulfillment. That wasn't what made her tick.

Only when she got out of the house and went back to school to get a degree in counseling did she begin to experience the fulfillment for which she was looking. My cousin finally understood who she was, what made her happy and what she needed to do to realize that happiness.

You, too, can find the kind of life that fits you best and then fashion that kind of life for yourself. Getting there is not difficult, but you must make some effort. Yes, you can find examples of people who just seem to have effortlessly fallen into a relationship that works. Perhaps they have found an ideal place to live. The feeling of ecstasy they experience daily convinces them this is where they will live forever. Usually these seemingly miraculous happenings have a pattern which spirals downward after reality sets in: annoyances pop up, problems and complications appear, unhappiness begins to infect the seemingly ideal situation and then, BOOM—divorce, relocation, job change.

Let's face it, impulsive decisions are romantic. But the important choices you make in your own life should fit you as well as a tailor-made suit. They must be shaped by what you know about your own strengths (and weaknesses) as a person.

Please don't misunderstand me. I am not promising you permanent and absolute happiness with ecstasy layered upon ecstasy every minute you live and breathe. Circumstances change, people change, organizations change. Your company may downsize. The economy may go into a long slump. Your mate may make some decisions which make it difficult for you to adapt. Or, you may tire of your career and want to start a new one.

This book cannot prevent your life from changing in ways that are sometimes unpredictable. But it can be there for you whenever you reach a point in your life where you need to rediscover yourself in order to make wise life decisions.

In any situation where you have to make important choices, the first step is to understand yourself. Having that knowledge helps define for you what steps you need to take to find the happiness, good health, wealth and wisdom which can be yours.

We're all different, and no single reaction is right or wrong. If you are going to take charge of your life, you have to know precisely what your likes and dislikes, strengths and weaknesses, needs and wants are. Why? Because that combination makes up who you are—your personality. The rest of this chapter will focus on a step-by-step procedure designed to reintroduce you to yourself and to record your findings. KEEPER #1—MY RESOURCES will be your written reminder of who you are, the resource that you will be drawing upon as you design your future.

Do not, repeat, do not try to anticipate what you will find. Just let the exploration process unfold, in order. Once you see and understand what you're dealing with—see yourself in a mirror as you truly are—you will be ready to make improvements in your life. Remember, by understanding yourself, you will learn to recognize how you are different from others and why the road you choose to follow must be unique. You will create your own pathway to happiness, good health, wealth and wisdom by using the resource that is *you*—by being yourself.

Step 1: Will the REAL YOU Please Stand Up?

OK, let's jump right in—it's time to take a <u>real</u> personality test. There are several such tests around that can give you an accurate picture of your fundamental traits and the principles that guide you, along with your other distinguishing characteristics.

If you have taken such a test in the past, you know that it will give you an accurate professional reading summarizing this special resource called *you.* Even if you disagree with parts of the analysis, the overall results will be helpful as you try to peer into the mirror to see who you are. The results will enable you to gauge your perception of yourself based on an objective professional opinion. This is more valuable than using your own subjective ideas or the negative feedback of someone you know.

The test included with this book is the Personality Analysis System (PAS). It's accurate, simple to use and easy to understand. There will be no head-scratching over how to use it. Also, it's not a test that will brutally beat you over the head making you feel you've been mugged. As the test's author, Dennis Drew, is quick to point out, "It is a POSITIVE ANALYSIS system which doesn't pull skeletons out of the closet."

The test is on the computer diskette accompanying this book. Most of you either have a home computer or have access to one through a friend, relative, or the public library. The 3 1/2 inch diskette containing the PAS is in two formats: the original DOS version and a Windows 95 version that you can use on any of the newer personal computers. Just follow the instructions on the diskette to install it.

The disk is shareware. You purchased it as part of this book package. You are allowed to use the program yourself or share it with friends. But, as with any shareware product, you may want to pay a fee and register if you're interested in the detailed instruction manual, the complete version of the program, telephone technical support, and new versions of the program when they come out. For your purposes here, the Shareware program itself is just fine.

RESOURCE BOX

> If you do not have a computer that will operate this disk, make a visit to your reference librarian and ask him or her how to access the website "www.drewsoft.com" on the Internet. You'll be able to download the Windows 95 Version and take the PAS test on the spot.

Let me make something very clear. YOU DON'T HAVE TO BE A COMPUTER WIZARD TO TAKE THIS VERY IMPORTANT STEP. All you need to do is answer honestly the 30-point response sheet on page 65 called "MY PERSONAL QUESTIONNAIRE." The computer will do the rest, and it will produce a five-page report that will describe your personality so accurately you may find it a little unnerving.

If you live in some remote area with access to neither a computer nor the Internet, send me your completed questionnaire along with an SASE and I'll see that you receive your personality report. I won't see the results. Those are confidential. I will simply make sure you get them.

OK, go ahead. Fill out the questionnaire, input your responses to the computer and then read over your printed results.

"The real voyage of discovery consists not in seeking new landscapes, but in having new eyes."
—Marcel Proust

MY PERSONAL QUESTIONNAIRE

Personality Analysis System Response Sheet

IMPORTANT: Please fill out ALL information.

Name:_____ Date: _____

Instructions: This response sheet is to help you better understand your personality. There is no way you can "pass" or "fail", because this is not a test. It is simply a tool to help further communications between you and your friends and family.

Below are 30 terms. By circling the numbers 1 through 5, indicate HOW WELL THE TERM DESCRIBES YOU AS A PERSON. Use the following as a guide:

1-Not very 2-Just a little 3-Somewhat 4-Ordinarily 5-Very

1. Calm......... 1 2 (3) 4 5
2. Kind-hearted.. 1 2 3 4 (5)
3. Industrious... 1 2 3 (4) 5
4. Careful....... 1 2 3 (4) 5
5. Agreeable..... 1 2 3 4 (5)

6. Persuasive.... 1 (2) 3 4 5
7. Demanding..... 1 (2) 3 4 5
8. Talkative..... 1 2 (3) 4 5
9. Modest........ 1 2 3 (4) 5
10. Generous..... 1 2 3 (4) 5

11. Spontaneous.. 1 2 (3) 4 5
12. Soft-hearted 1 2 3 4 (5)
13. Pleasant..... 1 2 3 (4) 5
14. Spirited..... 1 2 (3) 4 5
15. Attractive... 1 2 3 (4) 5

16. Fussy......... 1 2 (3) 4 5
17. Compassionate.. 1 2 3 4 (5)
18. Earnest....... 1 2 3 (4)(5)
19. Shy........... 1 2 3 (4) 5
20. Daring........ 1 (2)(3) 4 5

21. Persistent..... 1 2 (3) 4 5
22. Individualistic 1 2 3 (4) 5
23. Selfish........ 1 2 (3) 4 5
24. Compelling..... 1 2 (3) 4 5
25. Good-natured... 1 2 3 4 (5)

26. Understanding.. 1 2 3 4 (5)
27. Adaptable...... 1 2 3 (4) 5
28. Aggressive..... 1 2 (3) 4 5
29. Outgoing....... 1 2 (3) 4 5
30. Controlling.... 1 2 (3) 4 5

Please make sure ALL 30 terms are marked then enter the results into the PAS program.

What do you think? Is the person described in your PAS report the same one you see in the mirror? Go back and read it again. There's some important material there. Perhaps you have never read a report which spells out how you tend to act, how you make decisions, and what motivates or discourages you. The values and principles by which you live will also become apparent to you.

I know this is a lot to swallow in one sitting. So, after you've read the report once, maybe twice, put it down. Let it incubate for a day. Sleep on it until tomorrow. Then read through the report again and make out two lists:

1. The features describing you that you <u>agree</u> with.

2. The features describing you that you <u>disagree</u> with.

Now put these lists, one clearly marked AGREE WITH and the other marked DISAGREE WITH right next to your report. You'll need them in a few minutes.

Now, pat yourself on the back. You've just taken a giant step toward learning who you really are.

Step 2: Identifying the IDEAL YOU

If taking personality tests or looking at yourself in this way is brand new to you, you have just been introduced to a few terms that psychologists use when describing people. Acquiring a working knowledge of some of these terms will help you understand yourself even better. Since these terms will be used throughout the book, you need to become familiar with them.

- TRAITS are the personality characteristics you show by the way you act. For example, some people are daring, adaptable, sensitive, talkative or thoughtful—qualities demonstrated by the way they behave in their daily interactions with others.

- INTERESTS are simply activities you enjoy doing. They can include reading, watching TV, working out, dating or going on retreats.

- ROLES are the ways in which you act as you associate with and move among other people in a specified and defined manner. Roles can include being a friend, a coach, a student, or even a supermarket shopper. All require doing certain things and acting in certain ways.

- PRINCIPLES are the ideas that are most important to you. These concepts are your guiding stars, the values around which you base your life. Integrity, knowledge, moderation and making a contribution to the community, are some common examples.

● BELIEFS are groups of ideas that, when put together, define entire institutions, including such familiar examples as God, democracy, family, science and medicine, to name a few.

Look over these definitions and try to come up with some examples of your own. Look over your PAS report. There you will find examples of each of these terms that pertain directly to you.

So, if you had to make a list of the roles you play, the traits you display or the principles that guide you, you would understand what I meant, right? Well, if not, go back and look at those definitions again. Keep working on understanding them. You will be taking several steps on your journey to a new and happy life in which you will be putting these definitions to use.

On the next few pages you will find Table I which contains some examples of all these terms in the various areas of life. Remember, what you see here are only examples—your personality certainly involves characteristics that are not included in Table I.

Table I

Terms to Help You
Understand Your Personality

As a <u>unique</u> individual, you exhibit characteristics within five Areas of Life (Cultural, Mental, Physical, Social, and Spiritual):

TRAITS-personality characteristics that you display,

INTERESTS-activities that you choose to pursue,

ROLES-ways in which you interact with others,

PRINCIPLES-virtues that represent your "guiding stars," and

BELIEFS-institutional ideas about which you feel strongly.

Here are some <u>samples in each</u> category.

(TRAITS)

CULTURAL	MENTAL	PHYSICAL	SOCIAL	SPIRITUAL
Efficient	Intelligent	Coordinated	Sensitive	Intuitive
Responsible	Analytical	Strong	Influential	Principled
Productive	Precise	Fast	Agreeable	Calm
Adaptable	Organized	Attractive	Persuasive	Reflective
Industrious	Imaginative	Daring	Talkative	
	Logical		Selfless	

(INTERESTS)

CULTURAL	MENTAL	PHYSICAL	SOCIAL	SPIRITUAL
Watch TV	Read	Work out	Date	Meditate
Go school	Do Xword	Walk	Gatherings	Go to church
Go to movie	Take notes	Compete	Parties	Go on retreat
Housework	Study	Dance	"Hang out"	See nature
Drive car	Do research	Groom	Socials	Pray
Go to work	Surf "net"		"Do lunch"	Heal self
Buy things	Watch PBS			Keep diary

(ROLES)

CULTURAL	MENTAL	PHYSICAL	SOCIAL	SPIRITUAL
Employee	Student	Athlete	Friend	Soul Mate
Boss	Teacher	Jogger	Relative	Counselor
Shopper	Thinker	Coach	Spouse	Pastor
Investor	Scientist	Dancer	Acquan'ce	Artist
Entrepreneur		Swimmer		Medium
Vacationer		Eater		Psychic
Homemaker				

(PRINCIPLES)

CULTURAL	MENTAL	PHYSICAL	SOCIAL	SPIRITUAL
Industry	Learning	Activity	Trust	Service
Contribution	Sharing	Nutrition	Integrity	Reciprocity
Thrift	Knowledge	Rest	Caring	Devotion
Saving	Freedom	Moderation	Love	Beauty
Simplicity	Growth	"Your Best"	Humility	Harmony
Equality	Structure	Pleasure	Respect	Insight
Independence	Clarity	Safety	Cooperation	Morality
Quality	Challenge	Longevity	Fun	Creativity
Peace	Order	Well being	Fairness	
Security		Hygiene	Status	

(BELIEFS)

CULTURAL	MENTAL	PHYSICAL	SOCIAL	SPIRITUAL
Democracy	Education	Comp Sports	Family	God
Capitalism	Science	Medicine	Fraternity	Reincarnation
Country	ESP	Exercise	Reunions	Metaphysics
Currency	Human mind	Home	Justice	Religion
Insurance	*Intuition*	*Self Responsibility*		
Social Security				

Go ahead and add some of your own examples to the lists. Show yourself that you have a good feel for these terms.

OK, now that you're feeling comfortable with these definitions, you should get yourself into a reflective state of mind. Go someplace where you won't be interrupted for a few minutes. If you have kids in the house, wait until they go to sleep. Do whatever you need to in order to have a little peace and quiet and time to reflect.

Now that you won't be interrupted, imagine that you are attending your own funeral. Yeah, I know, it sounds morbid, but remember, you're just imagining here. Pretend that you've lived a long life and have been in contact with many people along the way. During those contacts, you've played a variety of roles. For example, you played the role of son or daughter to your mother and father. You may be a parent to your own children. You played the role of student to your teachers. You were an employee for all of the managers you worked for and possibly a supervisor or mentor for others. You have also been a friend, a good friend, to some special people.

Assume that you carried out each of these roles to the absolute maximum of your abilities. The people gathered to pay their respects would have *only praise* for you. Imagine what your mother, father, brother, sister, son, daughter, friends, teachers, managers, employees, and friends would say about your performance in those roles as they pay tribute to you and eulogize your life. Specifically, focus on the words they would use to describe the major character traits you displayed and the principles that guided the way you acted with them.

There's a form on page 75 on which you can make a list of as many roles as you can think of. These roles can be ones you've played in the past or ones you expect to play in the future. Next to each role, put the name of the individual, real or imaginary, who is making the tribute. In the next two columns record the major trait and principle that person highlighted in his or her imaginary tribute to you.

Don't zip through this one. Spend a few minutes steeping yourself in each role. Think about your interactions with that person and the <u>perception</u> that you and others had about how you acted in that role. When you were a student, were you logical and responsible? Talkative and competitive? Intuitive and eager? Were you driven by the principle of integrity? Making a contribution? Acquiring knowledge?

To give you a start, let me show you some of my entries.

ROLE	PERSON	TRAIT	PRINCIPLE
Son	My mother	Intelligent	Trust
Brother	My sister	Competitive	Thrift
Employee	My supervisor	Responsible	Service

If you're having a little trouble figuring out what kind of roles you play, mentally take yourself through an average week. Think of the people you frequently talk to, either in person or by phone, fax or Internet. Are you the relative of any of them? If so, what's your relationship? Brother, sister, daughter, mother, father? How about the people you relate to at work? Perhaps your relationship there is as a coworker, manager, subordinate or consultant.

How about the people outside of work? Neighbors, acquaintances and friends are all possibilities. How about many of the things you do during a week? If you go to the supermarket, the gas station, the dry cleaners, you're a customer. If you see someone in a professional capacity whether it's a lawyer or accountant, you're a client. And if you see someone in the medical arts, such as a doctor, dentist or acupuncturist, you're a patient. Make a list of the people you come into contact with over an average month, then concentrate on the really important ones for your pretend eulogy.

Again, this is not some morbid exercise. It is an excellent way for you to get in touch with the way others see you or at least the way you would like others to see you. Although it may appear to be somewhat idealistic, that's okay. At least it will give you some ideals to consider as you continue down the road of giving direction to your life.

On the next page record your summary of My Eulogy.

"Success always has been and always will be the natural result of what a man is; not what he pretends to be."   —Paul J. Meyer

My Eulogy—The Tribute to My Life

ROLE	PERSON	TRAIT	PRINCIPLE
Child	My Dad	Responsible	Service
Student			
Date			
Friend	Christine	Principled	Devotion
Employee	Bill R	Agreeable	Contribution
Wife	Treak	Loyal	Selfless
Sister	Neoma	Productive	Creativity
Friend	Lynette	Strong	Growth

NOTE: You can probably list 10 or 12 different roles that you've played or expect to play during your life. It's OK if you include more than one friend or teacher or supervisor, particularly if you think they perceive you as displaying different traits and principles. If you had any trouble coming up with adequate descriptions during this exercise, take another look at Table I. There you'll find a partial list of roles, traits, and principles to help you with your thinking.

And now, congratulations! Let your ego immerse itself in all this praise, like a gentle wave washing over you in the surf. You've just taken a big step toward making your life the fulfilling experience it should be. You have learned what your *ideal self* looks like. You've just let yourself put the best person you can be down on paper. This is how you would like others to see and remember you.

Take a few more minutes and look over the roles, traits and principles that you have recorded. They will turn out to be very important as you begin to use this new self-awareness to create your future of success and happiness.

RESOURCE BOX

If you have a good friend who you trust, he or she can be an excellent source of input about your personality. Just ask for feedback. You may also want to share your PAS Report and see if your good friend agrees with the description of you. Perhaps your friend will want to take the PAS Test. If so, you know the routine. Type in his or her responses and presto, out comes a five-page personality report. Comparing your similarities and differences with someone you know very well will reinforce in your mind what distinguishes you as a unique individual and help you discover who you really are.

Step 3: Putting the pieces of the puzzle together.

You've just completed another leg of your journey in this chapter. Look back at how far you've come in the process of understanding yourself. The hard work is over. You now have

- An image of the IDEAL person you would like to be,

- A description of the REAL you, and possibly

- Some supplementary feedback from others.

Now it's time to assemble all this information and create a profile of who you <u>really</u> are. Look at those two lists you put to one side after you completed your own PAS test. Those are the lists labeled "AGREE WITH" and "DISAGREE WITH." Now take another look at them and see if you want to make any changes.

Are there any items you disagreed with that you now see as being right, at least in part? Maybe you were too quick to agree to some items that you now think are not on target after all. Whatever the case, think things through in light of any discussions with a trustworthy friend and update your lists with your current thinking about what you are like.

Now you're ready for the final step of your self-discovery expedition. You need to summarize your current perception of who you really are in a way that is going to prepare you to create a new life for yourself.

At this point you are faced with an important choice.

1. You can continue with the life you have, or

2. You can leave behind the sadness, the frustration and the misery of the past when you were trying to be someone you are not.

To choose number two means you can embark upon creating a happy, fulfilling and joyful future for yourself by "living within yourself" and using your unique resources intelligently. When you have completed the form, "MY RESOURCES—The Highlights of My Personality," you will have formed the foundation upon which you can build your future.

Where is this sheet? It's on page 80 <u>and</u> in the KEEPER Forms Section, where it is also called KEEPER #1. You'll find a number of forms together there. They're all in the same place so that as you complete each step of the process of taking control of your life, you can find the really important forms easily. These forms, including The Highlights of My Personality, will help you to point your life in the direction that is right for you.

Once you've completed KEEPER #1—MY RESOURCES, you will have reached a major milestone—not just in this book, but in your life. Very few people ever reach this point of self-understanding and self-acceptance in their lives. But <u>all happy people</u> have passed this way.

They have been here because they know how important it is to understand themselves before they can have a life full of happiness, good health, wealth and wisdom. If you don't take the time to understand who you are and how you differ from other people—the individuality of your personality—then you will continue to be frustrated as you try to be someone else. You will have little chance to put your own strengths to work.

HOT TIP

If you want to be successful,
<u>use</u> your TALENTS.
If you want to be happy,
<u>accept</u> your LIMITATIONS.

KEEPER #1

MY RESOURCES

The Highlights of My Personality

My character strengths (traits) are

Fun   Loyal   careful
Creative   Strong   Supportive
agreeable   Responsible

My most significant limitations are

making decisions
communicating my thoughts

The activities I enjoy most are

laugh   things I'm good at
Reading   Parties   Retreat
Walking   Self care   good nutrition
play time

The roles I prefer to play are

Student   Artist
Teacher   Entrepreneur
Friend

My strongest institutional beliefs are

Self responsibility   metaphysics
Family   alternative med
Intuition   exercise

The most important principles that guide my life are

peace   Love   growth
Clarity   harmony   Service
friendship   Creativity

Now that you've finished answering the question "Who Am I?", you should be feeling a new sense of self-confidence and inner peace. You now know who you are. That is the first step in taking control of your life.

Are you ready to join the ranks of those who are happy and successful? If so, it's time to move on to the next question: "Why am I here?" After all, it's not much good to understand yourself if you don't define and shape how you want to use who you are. You will not be fulfilled until you use your valuable resources in the way most satisfying to you. Chances are that will happen when you are applying your strengths to play roles which benefit others. At the same time, you will be guided by the principles that are most important to you. Now, let's continue your journey.

Chapter 3

How to Discover Why You Are Here

People who are happy, healthy, wealthy and wise understand not only <u>who</u> they are but also <u>why</u> they are here—their missions in life. They use their personality strengths to play roles for the benefit of others while being guided by their own strong principles. By behaving in a manner consistent with their missions, such people enjoy life totally. They are doing what is really important to them and what is easy for them to do.

> "We make a living by what we get,
> We make a life by what we give."
> — Sir Winston Churchill

In this chapter you will learn how to create you own Mission Statements that explain why you are here. You will

- Step outside yourself to identify what's going on in the world that's really important to you.
- Focus on the most important roles you play that exercise your body, mind, emotions and intuition.

- Commit to live your life the way happy and successful people do—living up to your full potential while making a contribution to the lives of others.
- Summarize why you are here on KEEPER #2—MY MISSION STATEMENTS.

As with the other important Keepers, MY MISSION STATEMENTS can be found in the KEEPERS Forms Section. You can easily refer to "why you are here" as you continue your journey toward a rich, rewarding and fulfilling life.

Look at how far you've come already! You started not knowing who you really are, and now you do. Or at least you know a lot more about yourself than you did before. That's a huge achievement, and you should be proud of it.

You also know how you are different from everyone else—what makes you special, unique, what makes you...YOU. You know your strengths, your limitations.

Now it's time to put your newly won knowledge to use. There's no point in knowing who you are and the distinct ways in which you're different if you don't do something with what you know. Now it's time to figure out why you're here—what your mission is while you're here

Imagine how good you'll feel, how productive you'll be, how much happiness you'll have, knowing <u>exactly</u> what you're supposed to be doing. Imagine how much more fulfilled you'll be when you find out why you are here.

Don't worry, I'm not getting metaphysical on you. I'm not talking about some grandiose ambition such as finding a cure for AIDS. Your mission can be as simple and modest as using your talents and abilities to

- meet strangers in the park and make them laugh, or

- manufacture quality hand tools in your garage, or

- be a career homemaker for your family, or

- do the job you have or want to have with real service, devotion and passion.

Usually your mission is not your job. Repeat: Usually, your mission is NOT your job. It's the role or roles that you play which are true reflections of who you are. It's the things you do which combine your interests, traits, beliefs and principles. We will look into some of those in a moment. For now, just know that it is the ROLES that you play while expressing the PRINCIPLES that are the guideposts by which you conduct your life. Rarely does anybody have a job that lives up to that standard.

For example, suppose one of your major traits is the ability to get people to pour out their innermost thoughts and feelings to you. If one of your guideposts is the importance of accepting situations and enriching life with humor, then meeting people in the park to make them laugh could very well be why you are here.

I met such a man on a park bench in Victoria, British Columbia several years ago. He was friendly and he made me laugh. We talked about our lives and our hopes. He was truly content—and he had terminal cancer. Despite his illness he was one of the happiest people I have ever met. It was obvious to me he was fulfilling one of his missions in life. There he sat, wearing his joy for life like a cloak that he was anxious to share with anyone. We exchanged insights that day and I shall never forget him.

I'm not going to judge your missions in life and you shouldn't either. I simply want to help you discover why you're here and to accept the reasons for your existence. Why? So you can make happiness, health, wealth and wisdom a reality in your life.

Sounds overblown? Sounds about as trustworthy as a politician's promises the day before an election? Not so. Finding out your mission in life is something you can do easily. It's as simple as ABC if you'll just follow the step-by-step procedure in this chapter.

So, don't look to your friends, your companion, your mother or brother for the answer. The only place you'll find your missions is within yourself. The fun part about it is that your reasons for being here are as individual as a fingerprint. Your mission is yours alone. Nobody else has one quite like it.

> "Nothing
> can bring you peace
> but yourself."
> —Ralph Waldo Emerson

RESOURCE BOX

An excellent way to get in touch with what's important to you is to start writing in a journal — a Mission Workbook. A pocket-sized notebook from the drugstore will do. Get into the habit of spending <u>five minutes each day</u> recording your hopes and dreams for the future, your ideas for improving your life or something significant that happened in the previous 24 hours. Create a quiet place and time to write in your Mission Workbook <u>every</u> day. Although the results will not be immediate, they will be both life-changing and permanent when they eventually occur.

Now that you know who you are, discovering why you are here is relatively easy. You've done more than half the work already. For example, when my son was struggling at the age of 20 to discover his identity in life, he jumped from one interest to another. He never followed through on anything. But once he took a personality test and discovered who he is, he immediately began to envision why he is here. It was the logical next step in taking control of his life.

He is naturally intuitive and very sensitive to other people, but had been quite self-centered up to that point. After taking the personality test, he started to approach his relationships differently. He wanted to use his talents to help others by relieving their pain. When he embraced this idea as his mission, the rest of his life started to fall into place. Knowing why he is here gave him momentum to prepare for a career in physical therapy; he attracted an intelligent and compatible wife; his family relationships became enriching for all; and he found an inner peace which encouraged them to have children.

Your life, too, will take on much clearer definition when you discover why you are here. You will play the roles you choose to play for all the right reasons, not just for money or power or fame. Interestingly, when you are being yourself, you will find that you can have almost anything you want. If you want good health, it can be yours. If you want wealth, it can be yours. If you want wisdom, it can be yours. And if you want happiness, that can be yours as well.

Please recognize that you have not come to Lourdes. This book will not produce miracles just because you bought it. But if you follow the steps and be your self, it will bring out the best that is in you. Your life will become closer to what you have always wanted it to be.

> "You can have anything you want. You just can't have everything you want."
> —Peter McWilliams

So, don't wait another second. Let's get on with the business of finding out why you're here.

Step 1: What Are Your "Worthy Causes?"

With all of the introspection you've been doing, you may be tempted to try to forget that there is a whole wide world out there beyond yourself. Many of the current events in your newspaper or on the evening news have little or no direct bearing on your life. Even so, they're very significant to the lives of others.

Think about revolutions and elections, natural disasters and festivals, recessions and economic booms, death and medical breakthroughs, divorces and weddings, suicides and spiritual awakenings, career-ending disabilities and superhuman achievements. Yes, things are happening out there. Some good. Some bad. Some affecting you. Some affecting only others. Some you are indifferent to. Some you care about very much.

It's the last category, the ones you feel strongly about, that you should concentrate on now. We need to bring to your consciousness some of the human experiences that are outside of yourself, but are nevertheless important to you for one reason or another. Identifying such "worthy causes" will help you understand the principles most significant to you and the people who you believe need help. These elements are two of the ingredients of any Mission Statement.

To find out what these issues are, you need an overview of what's going on out there in the real world. Unless you have a month to go traveling and experience things firsthand, I suggest you spend an hour or so on one of two possible exercises:

1   Go out and buy a metropolitan newspaper and read it from cover to cover. I'm not talking about some 20-page local weekly you can leaf through in five minutes. I'm talking about a thick, multi-section daily covering local, regional, state, national, and international issues in depth and in detail. The *New York Times* and *Los Angeles Times* come to mind, but choose whatever metropolitan paper you can most conveniently locate. If you don't have a source nearby, make a trip to your local library and browse through your closest metropolitan newspaper Sunday edition. Find the one that interests you the most, and plan to spend a minimum of an hour with it. Or,

2   Sit and watch CNN news for a solid hour. Don't be passive, get involved in the issues. Empathize with those who are experiencing hardship and pay particular attention to the situations that stir strong feelings within you. Think about the problems big or small you feel need to be resolved.

RESOURCE BOX

If you are Internet literate, click on NEWS and spend your time exploring the top stories that command your attention. Allow yourself to become involved emotionally with the human or inhumane nature of issues being described.

No matter which alternative you choose, you will also need a pen and blank piece of paper at your side for this step. Title the blank sheet "My Worthy Causes." As you read the newspaper or get absorbed in the CNN News or uncover current issues on the Net, you will find yourself saying: "Something should be done about _____ _____." Make a list on your blank paper of those topics. To you, these topics are worthy causes—something that "somebody should do something about."

Finished? Okay, good job! You are now a step closer to being able to create your Mission Statements. You have identified problems that concern you, people who need help and principles that are important to you. Keep the "My Worthy Causes" list handy. You will be referring to it later in this chapter. These causes are an integral part of your journey toward a life of happiness and fulfillment.

Learn to Nurture Your Body, Mind, Emotions and Intuition

When you create Mission Statements, you are identifying the reason why you are here: the TRAITS you exhibit and the PRINCIPLES you live by transformed into action by the ROLES you play. That's right, the very same traits, roles and principles that appeared on My Eulogy and on KEEPER #1—MY RESOURCES. They also appeared in Table I where they were categorized into the five Areas of Life: physical, mental, social, spiritual and cultural.

Happy people live balanced lives in which they exercise all of their faculties—body, mind, emotions and instincts. Forgetting to nurture any of these human "parts" is unhealthy and can be a major source of frustration and dissatisfaction. The creation of your Mission Statements will give you an opportunity to increase your happiness in life by including roles that stimulate each of your faculties.

To do this, you need to be conscious of the five Areas of Life. You may already have noticed the connection among the <u>five</u> Areas of Life and the <u>four</u> faculties. Here's how it works:

- Physical (the playground for your body). This area is the one you can see, feel and touch. It is the most basic for your existence. It requires food, air, and water. It's also the area you think about when you are concerned with health and long life. Some physical roles you can play are as a person who performs, trains, relaxes, eats and exercises. Always you are primarily using your <u>body</u> when involved with physical roles.

Physical Area of Life

- Mental (the playground for your mind). This area primarily lives inside your head. It's the intellectual part of you. It focuses on learning, research, knowledge and education. Some roles you can play here are student, teacher, thinker, scientist or executive secretary. Each of these roles draws upon your <u>mind</u> as its <u>primary</u> resource.

Mental Area of Life

- Social (the playground for your emotions). This area represents your interaction, or lack of it, with others. It shows the extent to which you spend time, both with other people and alone. Some of your social roles can include being an acquaintance, friend, relative, spouse, lover, team player, or drinking buddy. Your <u>emotions</u> get top billing when you perform a social role.

Social Area of Life

- Spiritual (the playground for your instincts). When you are functioning in this area, you believe without having much, if any physical evidence to support your opinion. It includes such beliefs as God, reincarnation, the Buddha as prophet, voodoo, the inherent goodness of man, or spiritual healing. Many counselors, psychics, pastors, priests and even soul mates play spiritual roles. They are exercising their <u>instincts</u> when they put their faith in a particular belief system.

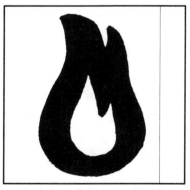

Spiritual Area of Life

- Cultural (the playground for your marketable skills). This is the area where you probably spend most of your time currently. It includes everything you do to make money, to buy material things, to travel from here to there and even to decorate your home. It also includes cultural diversions such as watching television. You are playing a cultural role when you are an employee, a shopper, a vacationer, a voter or a homemaker. In such situations, you are not exercising one of your four basic human faculties. Instead, you are employing

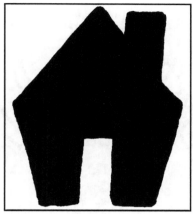

Cultural Area of Life

your marketable skills by working to acquire the cultural SYMBOLS of happiness and success: dollars or possessions or frequent flyer miles or pictures on the wall. To the extent that a marketable skill involves your body, mind, emotions or instincts, you may be operating in two or more Areas of Life. For example, a professional wrestler is clearly exercising his body at the same time he is earning a living playing this cultural role.

Understanding these categories will make it easier for you to nurture all of your faculties and create the underpinning of a balanced life. I will help you do this by focusing on your roles and principles in each area of life as you discover why you are here.

Remember, if you do a good job of understanding yourself and your mission in life, everything will start to make sense for you. You will do things in support of your missions and you will feel good about yourself as you begin getting whatever it is you want in life. Let's review how this happens.

Chart 1
How it Works

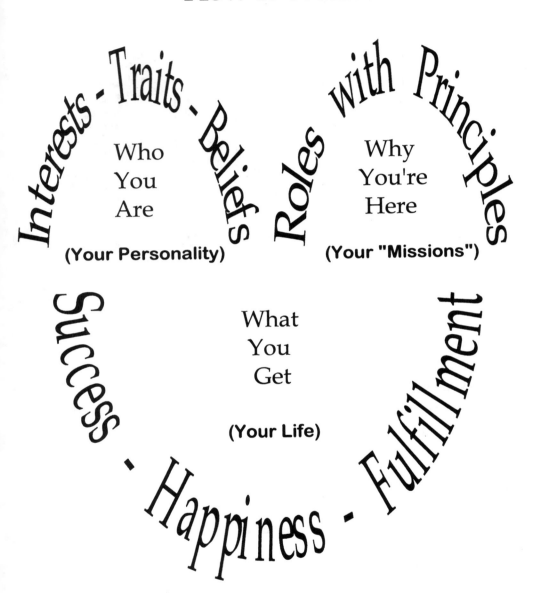

Interests - Traits - Beliefs

Roles with Principles

Who
You
Are

(Your Personality)

Why
You're
Here

(Your "Missions")

What
You
Get

(Your Life)

Success - Happiness - Fulfillment

Let me give you a personal example. One of my primary reasons for being here is to use my analytical abilities and organizational skills (TRAITS) to coach you (ROLE) so that I can make a significant contribution (PRINCIPLE) to your understanding of who you are and why you're here. When I'm involved in this cultural role, I am happy and at peace with myself. It gives me enormous satisfaction. When I succeed in this principled role, which is a true expression of who I am, I feel fulfilled.

Really, that's it. The whole story. It's just that simple. What this explanation should show you is how close you are to genuine happiness and getting the rewards you want. This is what you must do. Bridge the gap between WHO you are and WHAT you get. The bridge between "being" and "having" is understanding WHY you are here. So, you need to find out why you're here so you can build your personal bridge between who you are and what you get. The result will be the future of happiness, success and fulfillment that you know you deserve.

Step 2: Identifying Your Important Roles in Each Area of Life

When you were working on understanding yourself and you created KEEPER #1—MY RESOURCES, many traits, interests, roles, beliefs, and principles you listed were probably part of the CULTURAL slice of your life. Don't be surprised. As I mentioned, it's the part of your life with which you spend the most time. It's very natural to think of yourself as an employee, shopper or TV viewer, because you probably play those roles much more often than any others.

But don't neglect the other aspects of your life. You've got to nourish the physical, mental, social and spiritual parts of you as well. If you allow your body, mind, emotions or intuition to atrophy, you will not be in sync. Your health will suffer. Your attitude will turn negative. Your judgment will be cloudy. That is why it is so important for you to create Mission Statements involving all five Areas of Life.

Some roles you play clearly belong to one Area of Life. For example, as a student you are primarily involved in the mental Area of Life. You are spending most of your time exercising your mind. However, there is a social element based on your interaction and studying with other students. There is also a cultural aspect—the classroom experience plus all of the administrative details of registering, getting to and from class, and receiving a grade. Of course, these are minor compared to the primary focus of a student on the mental Area of Life.

Other roles may not be quite so clear-cut. For example, I sing with a barbershop quartet. You may view singing as a social role because of the interaction with three other people. Or, you may argue that it is a cultural role because there are organized practices to prepare for paid public performances. Granted, those are both aspects of the role but, for me, they are minor considerations compared to the overriding spiritual experience. I get into the songs intuitively using my instincts to feel the message of the composer through the melody, the harmony and the visual picture created by the words. For me, singing a four-part barbershop song is a spiritual role in which I impart to the listener the writer's intent.

If you play a role that involves two Areas of Life equally so that no one area is predominant, go ahead and categorize it in both areas. But most roles will emphasize a single area with just minor participation by some other Areas of Life.

Okay, you're ready to identify your most important roles in each of the five Areas of Life. My Mission Worksheet on the next page should be very easy for you to create after all the introspective thinking you did to create MY EULOGY and KEEPER #1—MY RESOURCES. This step involves selecting from the many roles that you identified on MY EULOGY, the most important role in each Area of Life.

If you can't decide between two social roles, put them both down. If you truly believe that one role is equally divided between two Areas of Life, enter it under both categories on the Mission Worksheet. If you find a blank Area of Life, you need to go back and review Table I (Terms To Help You Understand Your Personality). Do some creative thinking and come up with a future role that you would consider playing which fits that category. Remember, if you do not adequately exercise all of your basic faculties (body, mind, emotions and instincts) you will severely hinder your future of good health, wealth, wisdom and happiness.

"All my life I've always wanted to *be* somebody. But I see now I should have been more specific."
—Lily Tomlin's "Chrissy"

How to Be Happy, Healthy, Wealthy & Wise

My Mission Worksheet

AREA OF LIFE	MOST IMPORTANT ROLE	USING STRENGTHS (TRAITS)	GUIDED BY PRINCIPLES	FOR THE BENEFIT OF WHOM?
Physical	eating & exercise	attractive Enthusiasm coordinated	pleasure well being	myself & all I meet
Mental	Student teacher	patient thorough	learning & sharing	myself & my students
Social	friend	attentive	love	all I meet
Spiritual	Spiritual healer meditator	calm reflective	creativity harmony insight	friends family clients
Cultural	wife business owner employee	Responsible efficient adaptable	Security independence contribution	wife Patrick's students clients

PAYOFF BOX

Select one of your important roles that you haven't played for a while. Pick a time and place to act out this role during the coming week. TODAY, if possible. See how good and natural it feels to be yourself while you're helping others? Now put that role on your calendar again for next week. Remember, feeling good is one of the benefits of each step of the process.

Step 3: Letting Your Subconscious Help You

Up to this point in the chapter, you have taken several steps along the road to defining why you are here. They have resulted in your creating some personal documents which will be very useful to you in discovering your missions in life:

- Your Worthy Causes list,

- Your Mission Worksheet, and possibly

- Your Journal or Mission Workbook.

Now it's time to spend a few minutes reviewing these documents. Just find a quiet place where you won't be interrupted and read through this material you have created. Think about your hopes and dreams for the future, your self-improvement ideas, your strengths and principles in each Area of Life, and the worthy causes you have identified. If rereading these pages makes you feel relaxed, good. Don't fight the feeling. In fact, you should try to relax as much as you can while rereading what you have created. It will help open your subconscious to these ideas.

Try picturing yourself in a very peaceful setting—some place where you feel totally safe and secure and in touch with everything that's important. I find the image of a meadow with a quiet brook works for me. While absorbed in this serenity, imagine yourself playing your most important roles, using your strengths and being guided by your principles. Are you ready to commit to those ideals? Yes you are. To help make sure you're ready, repeat to yourself five times: *I will do everything in my power to live up to my potential.*

Now recall the worthy causes you identified when reading that metropolitan newspaper or watching CNN. Are you ready to commit to playing a role in some of those important causes? Repeat to yourself five times: *I will use my talents and abilities in a positive way to help others in need.* You should be feeling a kind of warm glow inside, a glow that echoes: "I will do good things with my life."

As you return from your relaxation state to your normal awareness state, you can be sure that your subconscious mind is now working on some mission statements for your conscious mind to consider. Don't worry. These statements may be incubating just below your consciousness right now, but they will emerge soon. And remember, by discovering why you are here, you will be well on your way to a rich and rewarding future.

Step 4: Unveiling Your Mission Statements

Brace yourself. It's time to reap the benefits of your efforts. You've taken some deep dives into both your conscious and subconscious levels to discover why you are here. Now it's time to write down your missions in life.

As you learned earlier, a meaningful mission statement has several components. It must address

- the traits and talents you will be using,

- the role that you will play,

- the principles that will guide your performance, and

- the people who will benefit from your efforts.

Looks like the information that's contained on My Mission Worksheet doesn't it? That's the major source! You've already done most of the work. All you have to do is transcribe the information.

Pages 103 and 104 contain a form on which you can record your mission statements. However, you will probably want to use KEEPER #2—MY MISSION STATEMENTS found in the KEEPER Forms Section. Then, you will have easy access to these important documents when you use them later to help you aim the future direction your life is going to take.

If you prefer to write your Mission Statements freestyle, that's fine. Just pull out a blank sheet of paper and write down why you are here. You need to state clearly and boldly the principled role that each mission represents. You must also list the strengths you will be using while helping others. These are your reasons for being here.

MY MISSION STATEMENTS

****

Using my _____, I will be a
　　　　　　　(traits and talents)

_____, guided by _____
　　　　(role)　　　　　　　　　　　　　(principles)

for the benefit of _____.
　　　　　　　　　　　　　(recipients)

****

Using my _____, I will be a
　　　　　　　(traits and talents)

_____, guided by _____
　　　　(role)　　　　　　　　　　　　　(principles)

for the benefit of _____.
　　　　　　　　　　　　　(recipients)

****

Using my _____, I will be a
　　　　　　　(traits and talents)

_____, guided by _____
　　　(role)　　　　　　　　　　　　　(principles)

for the benefit of _____.
　　　　　　　　　　　　　(recipients)

****

MY MISSION STATEMENTS (con't)

****

Using my _____, I will be a
                     (traits and talents)

_____, guided by _____
        (role)   (principles)

for the benefit of _____.
                          (recipients)

****

Using my _____, I will be a
                     (traits and talents)

_____, guided by _____
        (role)   (principles)

for the benefit of _____.
                          (recipients)

****

Using my _____, I will be a
                     (traits and talents)

_____, guided by _____
        (role)   (principles)

for the benefit of _____.
                          (recipients)

****

Let me give you another example of how a mission statement works. Before my cousin could make the transition from homemaker to guidance counselor, she not only had to understand who she is but also what she is doing here. It was during her reflective period of getting a Master's degree in psychology that she made the discovery. She said to herself something like this: "My mission is to use my intelligence and intuitive abilities (TRAITS) to counsel others (ROLE) with caring and humility (PRINCIPLES) to benefit friends, relatives, and students who need my help (RECIPIENTS)."

As you can see, this mission statement contains all the relevant ingredients:

1   It is a true reflection of my cousin's personality because it is based on her traits and talents;

2   It defines the principled role she will play, and

3   It identifies the beneficiaries of her actions.

Also notice that the statement is not confined to just one Area of Life. True, it includes the <u>cultural</u> area to the extent that it addresses the role of guidance counselor. But it also refers to roles in both the <u>social</u> area (because help is being offered to friends and relatives) and the <u>spiritual</u> area (using the broad interpretation of the term "counselor"). Only my cousin could tell us whether one of these areas is more prominent for her or whether two or more of the areas are significantly involved.

As you prepare your mission statements, you may find them limited to a particular Area of Life or you may find them overlapping two or more areas. Either way is fine. What's important is that you pin down in your own mind *my reasons for being here* and put those reasons on paper.

Don't feel you have to limit your missions to the important roles identified on My Mission Worksheet. Perhaps other missions will come to mind after meditating further on your Worthy Causes.

First focus on a role that you would consider playing. Then, identify the talents and traits that you would use as you perform this role. Third, identify the people who would benefit from your attention. Finally, specify the virtues that would guide you as you carry out this role. Be sure to use traits and principles that you have already identified as being basic to your very existence on KEEPER #1—MY RESOURCES. You see, this process builds on itself as you begin to customize your personal future. Your Mission Statements depend on your Resources. You are beginning to create your UNIQUE path to a life of fulfillment.

Don't skimp. Try to include at least one role from each Area of Life. The only way you're going to lead a well-rounded, full life is if you exercise all of your faculties: body, mind, emotions and intuition. Neglect one of the five areas and you will only move part way toward the happiness you deserve because your life will be out of balance.

For example, if the statement you read above were my cousin's only mission statement, she would need to prepare at least two more: one covering a role in the physical area and one for a role in the mental area. Knowing her as I do, I'm sure her physical mission reads something like: "using my inherent coordination and athleticism (TRAITS), I will play tennis (ROLE) with my friends (RECIPIENTS) to nurture our physical conditioning and good health (PRINCIPLES).

Don't worry, though, if you find that you're creating a large stack of mission statements. You can't have too many. There is no limit to the number of missions that you can choose to take on in your life. Each of your mission statements should be viewed as a map for your personal pathway—your future life of success and happiness.

As map makers learn more about the geography covered by their maps, the more detail they can show. Create your mission statements using a similar approach. Fine-tune them as you think them through individually and pay particular attention to their implications for you and your future. The more details you have, the clearer your pathway will be. Make your mission statements as clear as possible. Your happiness depends on it!

Although you may have been too busy to notice it, you have already begun to realize some benefits of knowing why you are here. You have increased your self-esteem. You now possess a new confidence that will aid you tremendously as you continue to turn your life around, pointing it in the direction you are defining.

Beware, though. Getting sidetracked is all too easy. Getting caught up in the personal agonies and problems of your cultural existence is not difficult. The result: you can let your mental, physical, social, and spiritual missions take a back seat. So, do a couple of things before you move on to stop yourself from indulging in your own pity party.

Memorize KEEPER #2—MY MISSION STATEMENTS. I can't impress upon you enough the importance of committing the details of your missions to memory. Only when your reasons for being here are as much a part of your life as your fingers, can you draw upon their power at any time and any place. Yes, any time and any place.

When you put down this book and go back out into the real world of school, work, relationships and competition, you must take along with you a working knowledge of why you are here. You can't just pat yourself on the back for making these discoveries. You need to begin making choices, taking action, and just plain living in accord with your mission statements. So, whatever it takes to memorize these things, now is the time to commit them to memory.

RESOURCE BOX

If you have a tape recorder, make a tape of yourself reading your Mission Statements in your most convincing voice. Try listening to the tape while driving in your car. This will help you memorize your missions and introduce your subconscious to the reasons why you are here. You will find it much easier to stay on track.

Do whatever it takes to internalize your missions in life and make them part of the very fiber of your being. Only then can you fashion a trail which will lead you to what you really deserve in life.

Look what you've accomplished! You have reached another major plateau on your journey. You may have noticed that this process gets a little tricky to navigate sometimes, but it does have plateaus on which you can rest. And, when you reach the top, you will have access to all the good things in life.

You aren't there yet, but you have positioned yourself to leave behind the sadness, misery, frustration, and despair of your past. You are now on the brink of a major breakthrough to a rewarding and satisfying life of success, happiness, and fulfillment that you deserve.

Now that you understand who you are and why you are here and have internalized this information, you are prepared to clear the way for the creation of your new existence. In Part 2, I will show you how to get rid of some obstacles that may be standing in your path. Even with the elements of your personal map in place, there still might be a little too much "clutter" in the way.

That's where Part 2 comes in. The next chapter will help you identify and clear away any fears or inappropriate excuses which may be standing in your way. Also, in Part 2 you will learn to explore some of the details of your current life. Then you can remove any complexities or imbalances standing in the way of your rebuilding project. If you "passed" Self-Tests #2 and #3 for those two problems, then you're ready to start walking your personal pathway right now. But don't kid yourself into believing you're ready to move on if you know you have obstacles standing in your way.

That's the purpose of Part 2: to clear away any debris, any obstructions, so there is room for you to give your life its new direction and meaning. You don't want any "demons" lurking about ready to attack you just as you are trying to take control of your life. So, if you need to eliminate some hangups or simplify your life first, then do it. I will show you how, step by step, in Part 2: Removing Obstacles from Your Life.

HOT TIP

A good plan today

is better than

a perfect plan tomorrow.

Part 2

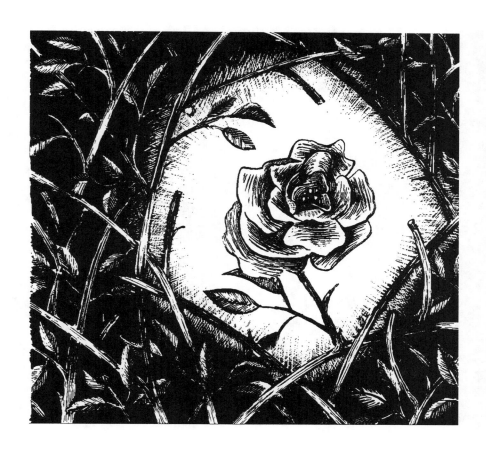

Removing
Obstacles from
Your Life

CHAPTER 4

How to Overcome Your Fears

> "We have met the enemy,
> and he is us."
> —Pogo

Harboring fears and hiding behind excuses are two of the most common reasons people remain stuck in their lives of unhappiness, frustration, depression, or worse. In order to grow and experience happiness, satisfaction, and fulfillment, you need to conquer your fears and shed all of those excuses for not taking control of your life. This chapter will help you put your fears and excuses behind so you can be *energized and open up new vistas* in your daily living.

To move toward those goals, in this chapter you will learn to

- Communicate with your subconscious mind (where all fears are rooted) by using an audio tape and tape recorder.

- Prepare an exhaustive list of your reasons for not having what you want. This list will show your REAL fears and allow you to get rid of excuses and artificial problems.

- Confront your "gremlins" by deciding what you need to do in order to overcome them; you will record these action items on KEEPER #3—MY "DO SOMETHING" IDEAS.

- Solicit the help of your subconscious by selecting a few substitute messages to counteract any fears that may be lingering there.

In this chapter, you will find and use the techniques that happy and successful people use to overcome their fears. They put a stop to excuses that have been standing in their way.

KEEPER #3—MY "DO SOMETHING" IDEAS is so important to your future that it is given a special place in the KEEPER Forms Section. There you will have easy access to it as you continue to give your life new meaning and structure during this journey of growth and self-improvement. If you need additional copies of KEEPER #3, tear along the perforated edge and duplicate it.

If you are seeking help in this chapter, it's probably because your Self-Test showed that you have some fears that are blocking your path to happiness.

Being afraid is okay. Honestly. It's part of the human condition. Some fears will preserve your life. You know that jumping from a plane without a parachute is not a good way to spend an afternoon. You know that trying to swallow a razor blade is going to hurt. So you're afraid to do those things, and you should be. Those fears will help keep you alive.

There are other fears, however, which get in the way of your happiness and success. You wouldn't be human if you weren't afraid of something at some point in your life. But the fears that hold you back get tangled up in your subconscious and set up housekeeping. And you know what? They'll live with you for the rest of your life unless <u>you</u> do something to evict them.

Excuses for not getting a grip on your fears are just as common as the fears themselves. Excuses go hand in hand with fears. As you struggle to deal with whatever terrifies you, your conscious mind devises reasons that you <u>should not do anything that might trigger one of these fears.</u> You'll start asking yourself questions such as "What if this" or "What if that happens?" Such excuses will paralyze you like a deer caught in a car's headlights and keep you from taking action.

Excuses are perfectly natural also. Don't feel guilty or inadequate or inferior when you have these thoughts and feelings. Just recognize that having them makes you human. That's the good news.

The bad news is that you will <u>never</u> be happy unless you deal with these issues. Being afraid may be human. Piling up excuse after excuse so you don't have to do something about your fears may be human also. But to make your life truly happy, you must not only understand yourself and your reasons for being here, you must also confront the fears and excuses that stand in your path.

For example, one of my clients, who is well educated and widely experienced in business, finance, marketing, counseling and communications, has a fear of specialization. "Jerry" hates the idea of focusing on one of his areas of expertise and letting go of the other ones for any length of time. The result: He is paralyzed and makes no real progress in any of his many talents. He will never achieve the success, fulfillment and happiness that he desires until he faces up to that fear.

But Jerry won't confront it. Instead, he dabbles in a host of entrepreneurial ventures. He bounces from one to another like a rubber ball off a hard wall without following through on any one of them. Consequently, he will never be satisfied with a "job well done" because he doesn't stick with one thing long enough to achieve any results. Then he complains loudly because he is

- not accomplishing anything,

- not making much money

- not putting money away for the future.

The sad part is, Jerry knows that his problem is the fear of specialization. He refuses to specialize anyway. Why? He keeps wondering aloud about any number of "What ifs?" What if he does specialize and loses a chance to make money on one of the projects he's dropped? Or misses something interesting because he let a project drop? Or he makes the wrong choice and one project he drops turns out to be more rewarding than the one he chose?

So, he lets all of his "what-iffing" paralyze him. The truly sad part—are you ready for this?—he remains dissatisfied and unhappy despite the fact that he

1   understands himself quite well. In fact, he has taken several personality tests, received counseling and can recite his strengths and weaknesses with great eloquence;

2   possesses an excellent grasp of what his mission is—he uses his talents, abilities, and general knowledge of life situations to help others make progress toward their hopes and dreams with great patience and selflessness;

3   lives a simple life with few material possessions, has few personal long-term commitments, and has only basic needs that are well within his means to satisfy.

Even though Jerry does many right things, he will die a bitter and frustrated man unless he confronts his fear of specialization. Only then will he be able to figure out how to make a commitment that will enable him to establish goals for himself. He can then follow a plan of action using all of his self-awareness, high principles, and tremendous potential.

So what's the "good" news?

If you resemble my client in any way, this description of his problems may make your life seem pretty bleak. Well, it should. If you're like Jerry, you're letting your fears stop you in your tracks. Major segments of your life may be closed off because of your fears. And those same fears could be robbing you of rich opportunities to be fulfilled. If you find yourself wandering around saying "What if this" or "What if that," then you have the same disease as my client.

The disease wears many disguises, but once you strip them away, the same ugly gremlin lurks underneath. If you fear the unknown (like my hometown baseball idol who has remained "stuck" all these years), you may be asking yourself, "What if I move and I'm not happy?"

You may fear change the same way many of my career counseling clients do. They want me to tell them that the jobs they have are the correct jobs for them. You might be asking as they do, "What if I change jobs and then my interests change. Won't I be unhappy?" Or, "What if this change makes my life too stressful?"

You may cringe at the prospect of failure like my client who refuses to establish goals for herself. Then you may ask, "What if I don't succeed and have to suffer all the humiliation of people seeing I didn't do what I said I would do?" Or, "What if I expose my real self and people don't like me anymore?"

That's right—fears and excuses will definitely stand in the way of your progress toward anything worthwhile. They will deprive you of the happiness, good health, wealth and wisdom that you deserve.

There is good news, and it's this simple: You (yes, you) can destroy the gremlin. You don't need hours and hours of expensive therapy sessions. You can conquer your fears and put an end to those "what if" questions ALL BY YOURSELF. That's what I will help you do, step by step, in the rest of this chapter.

By the way, this procedure is not based on some dramatic scientific breakthrough. It's really very simple and something you may have had some personal experience doing already.

I have. When I was a small child, my family lived in a two-story house with a basement. That basement was dark, with too many creepy corners we couldn't see into. In the cellar was a water pump which made eerie sounds and a coal furnace that made bellowing and grating noises which made my body shiver. Then there was the dank little room with the squeaky door where the coal was kept.

Let's face it, this place was a Halloween heaven but a little boy's nightmare. I can remember often charging up those cellar stairs scared out of my wits and shaking with fright. I didn't know if it was a monster or the bogeyman or what it was, but I was too frightened to stick around to find out. I was petrified of the dark.

Of course, being afraid of the dark is a very common fear among youngsters. Fortunately, my parents insisted that I go down to the basement to get them something on a number of occasions. They always assured me that there was nothing alive down there except me. I went down—and returned in one piece! Gradually I began to overcome my fear of the dark. (Although, I can still remember getting "twinges" of fright entering or leaving a dark area as a young adult.)

The moral of the story is simply this: My fear of the dark was overcome by repeatedly confronting what I thought was the bogeyman and never getting hurt. Each time I went into that cellar and returned safely, my *subconscious* mind became a little more convinced that there really <u>wasn't</u> anything to be afraid of. Repetition, repetition, repetition, and finally, the fear was conquered. What also disappeared (along with my fear of the dark) were all those excuses I used to have for not going down to the cellar in the first place. I just didn't need them anymore.

Do you know how good it feels to dump a fear? It's like removing a huge, heavy, fallen tree from your pathway so that you can continue your journey. The act generates self-confidence, fills you with a new sense of hope that you can do what you want to do, and energizes you to expand your life in new directions. That's why it's so important that you deal with your fears one at a time and put them behind you.

If you don't unshackle yourself from your fears, you are ruining your chances of ever taking charge of your future. Remember, you want to clear away some clutter in your path so you can keep traveling on the road you're building for yourself. As rewarding as finding and creating the road you want to travel may be, it is only a start. You have to actually travel that road to get where you want to go.

Step 1: Communicating with Your Subconscious

As you already know, fears are rooted in your subconscious. Naturally, the way to deal with those fears is to communicate with your subconscious. We did some of that in the last chapter when you were discovering your mission. As you recall, your subconscious mind gives and receives information best when you are in a very relaxed state.

To help put yourself in such a state, you need to create a personal tape recording using an audio tape. The tape will be a message that you'll listen to as you begin the process of overcoming your fears and excuses. The cost is cheap. If you don't have one, all you need is an inexpensive portable tape recorder and a 60-minute tape. They run between $10-$15.

You will also need a source of relaxing music (radio or CD). Choose whatever is the most soothing to you. You may prefer classical, instrumental, adult contemporary or country music. Be sure to select something that does <u>not</u> grab your attention. You'll be using it as pleasant background music intended to help you relax.

At this point, you also need to refer to Appendix A—The Pathway to Your Subconscious on pages 358-360 (these pages are perforated for easy removal and reference). They contain the message to read into your tape recorder creating Your Relaxation Tape. A watch or clock which keeps track of seconds will also come in handy.

Finally, you will need your fistful of mission statements (KEEPER #2 in the KEEPER Forms Section). Because you will be reading these descriptions of what you are doing here, make sure every statement is clearly legible if you haven't memorized them by now. In fact, if your missions in life are not firmly implanted in your memory, this is the perfect time to take a few minutes and MEMORIZE YOUR MISSION STATEMENTS!

Okay, you're all set. Put the 60-minute tape in your recorder. You'll need only Side A here. Using a compact disc or stereo or whatever you have, play the "mood music" you've selected. Let the tape record the music for a minute or so as you get ready to read The Pathway to Your Subconscious found in Appendix A into your recorder. Read in your most deliberate manner and your most soothing tone of voice. Take your time. Speak as though you are delivering a very special message to someone you really care about. But, just read it. You'll have plenty of opportunity to use your tape in a few minutes.

Don't be afraid to pause after each sentence. That short pause will give the message a good chance to sink into your mind when you are listening to it. Pause even a little longer between paragraphs, as the subject matter shifts. And be sure to honor all of the PAUSE instructions as you read The Pathway to Your Subconscious. Please note, you're not supposed to read the CAPITALIZED PHRASES aloud. These are instructions for you to follow in making the recording. Read everything else as written directly into the tape recorder.

When you are reciting your Mission Statements, it doesn't matter whether you have only one, three or a dozen. Recite the Mission Statements into your tape recorder at the appropriate places. If you have to read your statements (shame on you), go ahead, but you really need to memorize them if you're ever going to start realizing their benefits—a life with direction and focus.

The whole process of creating Your Relaxation Tape shouldn't take you much more than 30 minutes. After you've finished recording the tape, take a break. You'll need it. Listening to your tape will take you another 30 minutes and you'll be using a new state of mind.

RESOURCE BOX

If you have trouble working with a cassette tape recorder or don't like the sound of your own voice, you may want to recruit a close friend to prepare your tape. This option may be especially appealing if you have already been working with a friend on the Personality Analysis System in Chapter 2.

Listening to Your Relaxation Tape requires that you do just one thing: -------*relax*-------. So, find yourself a quiet, comfortable place where you won't be disturbed for 30 minutes and get on with it. If the telephone could be a problem, turn off the bells and let the answering machine take any calls. No answering machine? Unplug the phone or leave it off the hook or smothered in a pillow. If someone tries to reach you in the next 30 minutes with something really important, he or she will call back later. If the doorbell could be a problem, put a note on the door "GONE FISHIN'—BE BACK TOMORROW."

I think you get the point: This next 30 minutes must be completely uninterrupted, so do whatever is necessary to make that happen. Now rewind your tape to the beginning, sit yourself down in your favorite chair, and push PLAY.

> "The unexamined life
> is not
> worth living."
> —Socrates

Step 2: Open a Whole New World of Possibilities — Identify Your Fears and Excuses

Once the tape recorder finishes playing Your Relaxation Tape, congratulate yourself. You have just taken a giant step toward gaining control of your life. You have effectively communicated with your subconscious about your fears and excuses. In the process, your primary current fears have surfaced to your conscious mind where you can deal with them. Plus, you have committed the power of your subconscious to taking action against those irrational fears.

It's true. These developments will make sure that you are driving those gremlins, your fears, out of your path. If you continue your assault on them, they will not be obstacles to your future happiness much longer.

At this point, your current fears and excuses should be in the forefront of your mind. So, take out a sheet of paper and title it MY REASONS FOR NOT HAVING WHAT I WANT. Now, write down as many of your fears and excuses as you can think of. Don't try to prioritize them, just list them as they come to mind. It doesn't matter whether they are big concerns or small ones, just write them all down.

Have you finished the list? Are you sure? Look it over. Here is a list of some common fears people encounter. Should any of these fears be added to your list?

SOME COMMON FEARS

Failure	Not being in control emotionally
Public Speaking	Meeting & interacting with people
The water	Not being perfect
Flying	Specialization
The unknown	Taking tests
Dying	Making decisions
Change	Not having enough money
Cancer	Going to the dentist (doctor)
Making mistakes	Showing your feelings
Animals or insects	Being a victim of a violent crime

Again check your reasons for not having what you want. If your list still seems a little short, you might try listening to Your Relaxation Tape again. Sometimes your subconscious can be a little stubborn in relinquishing its deep dark secrets. So, try it again. You can use it as often as you like—after all, you did invest some time and effort into making it in the first place.

Okay, happy with the size of your list? Then take a deep breath, relax, and then read over what you've written. You'll find that some of these reasons are REAL fears like the ones on the list above; others are just excuses or imaginary limitations that you have grown accustomed to imposing on yourself. For example,

- a fear of failure is a REAL fear. But, the attitude "I won't even try because I can't do anything right" is just an excuse for you not to take action. Of course you do things right—you can tie your shoelaces can't you?

- a fear of public speaking is a REAL fear, but the attitude "I can't speak in public because my mouth gets all dry" is just an excuse not to take action. You've seen a lecturer take a drink of water.

- a fear of taking tests is a REAL fear, but the attitude "I can't go back to school because I don't have enough money" is an excuse not to take action. Student loans are a reality these days.

As you can see, excuses are your justifications to avoid taking action because of some underlying fear. Be sure to understand the difference.

Now go through your list of reasons one by one and cross out your EXCUSES—problems you know you can solve if you really want to. They are just rationalizations that you have been hanging on to or explanations that others will accept for your not taking action. But, you know they are not the REAL problems. Your fears living in your subconscious are the REAL problems.

SOME COMMON EXCUSES

Excuse for Not Taking Action	Possible Underlying Fear
I don't have time to do it well	Specialization
I am too old	Change
I am too young	The unknown
I am not smart enough	Taking tests
It's too hard	Not being perfect
My family has never done it	Failure
I might get hurt	Showing your feelings

After crossing out your excuses, take another piece of paper and title it MY REAL FEARS. Now transcribe each fear that remains on MY REASONS FOR NOT HAVING WHAT I WANT on to your new list of REAL fears. But as you write down each of these fears, ask yourself one more time, "Is this a REAL fear or just an excuse for not taking action?"

HOT TIP

A fear of making decisions is a REAL fear, but the attitude "I like to wait and see what happens first" is an excuse not to take action.

Make sure that you have transcribed only REAL fears like the ones on the table of SOME COMMON FEARS. Also make certain that you have crossed out all the problems that you already know how to handle. Then, take your first list and tear it up!

By doing so you will have taken care of, once and for all, those excuses, imaginary limitations, and artificial barriers that have been standing in the way of your life of happiness, success, and fulfillment. You have just taken some real action to get rid of these problems—you've destroyed them. How?

1   You crossed them out since they aren't REAL problems.

2   You discarded them and eliminated them from your life.

Your subconscious mind will do the rest. It will make sure that these excuses will not plague you anymore. And by removing them from your path, you have cleared the road you want to travel of some major obstructions. Now you're more ready than ever to move your life ahead along the path that you choose.

"Whether you think you can or not, you are right."
—Henry Ford

Step 3: Energize Yourself: Tackle Your REAL Fears

Fears are not only irrational and rooted in the subconscious, but are also based on ignorance. My fear of the dark when I was a child was based on the assumption that there really was something down in that cellar that was "going to get me." My assumption was wrong! I was ignorant about the facts of the situation.

When you are ignorant about something, you need to be educated. You need to learn the truth so you can make the correct assumptions. Correcting your misinformation at the conscious level will go a long way toward eliminating your fear.

RESOURCE BOX

Choose an "education method" that works for you. Don't overlook an alternative you've never tried before. For example,

- talk to a friend,

- read a book,

- take a class, or

- watch a PBS-TV program.

If you have a fear of making decisions, for instance, you need to find out everything you can about how to make decisions easily and correctly. Ask your reference librarian to point you in the direction of books that might explain how to do it. Talk to people who find decision-making easy and pick their brains. See what courses are available at your local community college on the subject.

In short, get prepared by learning how to do it right. This new knowledge will definitely increase your confidence that you can succeed. However, these "passive" educational techniques will only get you so far. You can't analyze something to death.

For example, my client who has the fear of specializing and has essentially handcuffed himself by giving in to this fear, has been educating himself for years. He has gone to workshops, read all the books, personally talked to the experts, and researched his options on the Internet. Even so, he's still searching, keeping his options open, refusing to make a choice because he's afraid specializing will cause him to miss a better opportunity. His rationalization—his excuse for not taking action—is, "There is a right answer and I'll wait until I find it."

There's another step to his education he hasn't yet tried. He hasn't really tried to find out what will happen when he looks the gremlin in the eye by DOING something. For him to do something means he must immerse himself in one of his specific interests—whether it's marketing, communications, finance or counseling.

He must commit to one of those projects and drop the others for some trial period of time, maybe a year or two. Until he does this, until he attacks his fear of specialization by taking an "active" approach, the gremlin will keep its stranglehold on his life.

My client is not alone. You, too, may be stuck in a bog of inactivity allowing one of your fears to control your life. DOING SOMETHING is probably the most effective way you can kick those gremlins, those irrational fears, out of your way.

> "Insanity is doing something the same way over and over, and expecting different results."
> —Alan Gasper

Talking to others, reading a book, watching TV, and taking a class are all passive approaches. But DOING SOMETHING will grip you mentally, physically, emotionally and intuitively. What you learn will come from what you do, not what others say you ought to do.

To help impress upon you the value of DOING SOMETHING to educate yourself about your fear, let me give you a personal example of a fear that I've shared with many—*public speaking*. You may already know that speaking in public petrifies people more than anything else. It's more widespread than the fear of heights, the fear of flying or even—believe it or not—the fear of death. This fear clutters the lives of more people than any other single fear. It was certainly an obstruction in my life for a long time.

When I was in my twenties, I was exploring many possible careers. My almost paralyzing fear of speaking in public throttled any thoughts about numerous careers. I immediately scratched off politics, law, teaching, sales, or management without a second thought. My excuses were

● politics is too crooked;

● law is too bureaucratic;

● teaching doesn't pay enough;

● sales work is too competitive.

Now I look back and see all too clearly that it wasn't my high principles, strong character or personal needs that caused me to dismiss any thoughts of those four careers. It was my raw and very real fear of public speaking.

I was letting this gremlin control and frighten me into taking technical career paths such as math, computers, engineering, and management science. None of these fields required much public speaking. Only when I decided, years later, that I really wanted to teach, did I have to face the utterly unpleasant reality of my fear.

Sure, I had made the occasional presentation during my years in business management and public administration. But it was usually addressing a group of people I knew about a project with which I was totally familiar. Even then, I would sweat and agonize over what I would say. I would try to second-guess every conceivable concern or objection. I would practice in front of a mirror, reviewing my choice of words repeatedly to make sure what I said would come out perfectly.

Even so, on the day of my talk, when I should have been feeling the supreme confidence of being prepared to the max, I would be a wreck. Two minutes into the presentation, beads of sweat would pop out on my forehead. Before long, streams of perspiration would be running down my face, back and sides. My throat would become dry and scratchy. My face would flush, my knees would wobble. To say I was scared, states it too lightly—fear almost turned me to stone!

Needless to say, I subjected myself to this torture as infrequently as possible. For 15 years I continued to shy away from projects, jobs, and positions in which public speaking was more than an occasional requirement. The gremlin was alive and kicking.

It wasn't until my mid-life switch into teaching that I finally took the time to educate myself about my fear of public speaking. I had to do it mostly out of desperation. I had grown weary of all the bickering and political maneuvering that were ingrained in the large organizations where I had been working.

I wanted to try my hand at teaching. The value of education had always been one of my strongest beliefs. Informally teaching others in some form or fashion always came naturally to me.

But, I was still plagued by my fear of public speaking. To overcome my ignorance of what public speaking is all about, I took a few classes and observed the different styles teachers used. I spoke with a few of them. I even read a couple of books on the subject. Was I ready? No way! I still needed to DO SOMETHING to complete my education.

So, while keeping my full-time job, I tried teaching an evening class in accounting one night a week. Once again I equipped myself to face down the gremlin. I prepared

- transparencies outlining my lectures,

- word-for-word notes of what I would say,

- examples all worked out in advance, and

- material for guest speakers to handle.

And you know what? I was just as scared as ever. My knees wobbled. My throat dried. My clothing was soaked with sweat. But I DID IT! I did it for ten grueling weeks. And by the time I finished, I had learned a few things. I learned:

1   There was no gremlin ready to humiliate me in public when I said something inelegantly or put the accent on the wrong syllable. No one was lurking in the hallway just waiting to jump out, pointing a finger and making me out to be a fool. In front of me were simply students interested in learning some material that I already knew.

2   Being the authority on a subject for a group of people is not intimidating as long as I stayed prepared and kept myself a step ahead.

3   Even in a group setting, I don't have to treat everyone in the same way. It's okay to relate to different personalities using different styles of my own. Students and other observers will accept and respect my behavioral differences.

In short, by DOING SOMETHING which confronted my gremlin head on, I learned that classroom teaching was something I really enjoyed doing. Once I discovered that fact, my fear of speaking in public was a thing of the past.

Ditching my gremlin opened up a whole vista for me, one which I had previously run from in fear. I have now completed 20 years of teaching, and I am still discovering new opportunities for fulfillment in my life through my cultural mission as a classroom instructor.

If I had not DONE SOMETHING to overcome my ignorance and fear, I might still be running from my personal gremlin. I would be afraid to open my mouth at a gathering of more than two people. I would be afraid that someone might think I was an idiot.

Are you ready to remove the unnecessary obstacles from your life? Are you ready to look your gremlin squarely in the eye? Then DO SOMETHING to confront your fear. You know what to do. Find KEEPER #3—MY "DO SOMETHING" IDEAS on page 136 and record each fear that you have identified. Also, write down a possible course of action to attack that obstruction to your life of happiness. I'm not asking you to carry out your ideas at this point. Just list some <u>active</u> ways in which you can energize yourself by overcoming the fears that are standing in your way.

These ideas are so important to your future happiness that they belong on KEEPER #3—MY "DO SOMETHING" IDEAS to confront my fears. Recording them in the Forms Section will give you quick access when you are ready to incorporate some of these ideas into your plans for the future. In <u>this</u> future, you are in control, not the gremlins.

KEEPER #3

MY "DO SOMETHING" IDEAS
To Confront My Fears

****

To overcome my fear of _____, I could

_____.
(possible course of action)

****

To overcome my fear of _____, I could

_____.
(possible course of action)

****

To overcome my fear of _____, I could

_____.
(possible course of action)

****

To overcome my fear of _____, I could

_____.
(possible course of action)

****

MY "DO SOMETHING" IDEAS (cont)

****

To overcome my fear of _____, I could

_____.

(possible course of action)

****

To overcome my fear of _____, I could

_____.

(possible course of action)

****

To overcome my fear of _____, I could

_____.

(possible course of action)

****

To overcome my fear of _____, I could

_____.

(possible course of action)

****

To overcome my fear of _____, I could

_____.

(possible course of action)

Step 4: Build Self-Confidence: Get Your Subconscious Involved

Let's see what you've accomplished so far in overcoming your fears and excuses for not taking control of your life. You have successfully

- communicated with your subconscious mind using your tailor-made Relaxation Tape,

- commissioned your subconscious mind to identify your fears and excuses so that you may have the freedom to be the best that YOU can possibly be,

- eliminated your excuses for not taking action,

- begun to educate yourself regarding your REAL ignorance-based fears.

Depending on how largely your gremlin looms in your path, this education process may take some time. My fear-of-public-speaking gremlin took several weeks to die. So remember this: You need to be both patient with yourself and persistent in your efforts.

> "Be not afraid of growing slowly, be afraid of standing still."
> —Chinese proverb

I did not push myself to make my fear and quaking go away in a day. Or even a week. I knew that I was facing my fear, and I knew that eventually it would get out of my way. Too many people beat up on themselves for not being perfect or, when they're trying to fix themselves, for not getting fixed fast enough.

Beating up on yourself will only cause you pain. Instead, brace yourself with the knowledge that your facing the fear will eventually force it to retreat. If it takes weeks or months, so be it. Your gremlin probably took years to grow if it looms so large in your life. Well obviously, it won't lose its grip, won't step out of your way, by tomorrow. Give it time. Even better, give yourself time. You deserve it.

You need to do one more thing to punch this process into high gear. Once again, you need to call upon your subconscious mind for assistance. Remember, your subconscious does not pass judgment. It accepts whatever you tell it as THE TRUTH and helps you make that truth actually happen.

If you tell your subconscious dark and ugly things about yourself or the world (say, for instance, that an evil beast is lurking in the cellar), you will behave as though what you've told your subconscious is TRUTH. (So whenever you're in the cellar you will run up the stairs trembling like a leaf in a windstorm so you can escape the beast.)

On the other hand, try talking nicely to your subconscious. If you feed it positive thoughts ("I will face each of my fears and excuses so that I may live an energized life open to new and rewarding experiences."), you will behave in a way to make that TRUTH come true. (You will enthusiastically educate yourself about your ignorance-based fears.)

It's up to you. If you choose to think dark and gloomy thoughts, your subconscious will help you create a dark and gloomy life. If you bring your thoughts out into the warmth and sunshine, you can make truly remarkable things happen in your life. This is the power of the subconscious, power which happy and successful people draw upon every day. We will be using this power again later as we construct your future of happiness, good health, wealth and wisdom in the next chapter.

For right now, program your subconscious to hit the accelerator and speed up the process of educating yourself regarding your ignorance-based fears. The keys to this programming are 1) **substitution** and 2) **repetition**.

If, for example, your gremlin is the fear of meeting and interacting with strangers, you need to give your subconscious mind a substitute message. That message must be positive and you must use it to replace your negative thoughts. For example, you could tell your subconscious:

- I am totally at ease when I am around other people;

- I am confident that each person I meet is a potential friend;

- Others enjoy my company and look forward to seeing me.

Using your conscious mind, choose the one or two substitute messages you want to use to replace your fear of being with strangers. Then repeat this thought to yourself. Repeat it frequently, particularly when you are relaxed and your subconscious is totally open to suggestion.

A very good time to deliver these substitute positive messages to your subconscious is just before you go to sleep at night. Repeat the message to yourself six or eight times. Before long, your subconscious will be working just as hard as your conscious mind to put that gremlin in its place. It will be out of your way and out of your life forever.

Table II beginning on the next page contains "Some Common Fears and Substitute Messages for Your Subconscious." Check to see if any of the fears on your list of MY REAL FEARS are included in Table II. If they are, consider programming your subconscious using some of these suggested positive messages. Feel free to create your own <u>positive</u> messages for these or other fears that you want to conquer.

> "The light
>
> of understanding
>
> dissolves
>
> the phantoms of fear."
>
> —Ellie Harold

Table II

Some Common Fears
with
Substitute Messages for Your Subconscious

Fear of Failure

- I have more faith in myself than ever before.
- I trust my judgment to do my very best.
- I can picture my project completed to my satisfaction.

Fear of Not Being in Control Emotionally

- The more irritating a situation becomes, the more patient and peaceful I will become.
- I am always in control because I can instantly see both sides of an issue.
- I am calm and secure because I know that I am responsible for my own emotions.
- The angrier other people are, the more relaxed I become.

Fear of Public Speaking

- I am calm and relaxed when I am called upon to speak in public.
- I enjoy speaking in public and my words flow smoothly and logically.
- My skin is dry, my mouth is moist, and my legs firm as I speak clearly and effectively in public.

Fear of Not Being Perfect

- I am secure and confident in my roles and activities.
- I accept myself as a positive, helpful, and loving person.
- My subconscious helps me to be the best that I can be.
- I can see my assignment completed to my satisfaction and I am ready to begin another.

Fear of Meeting & Interacting with People

- I am totally at ease when I am around other people.
- I am confident that each person I meet is a potential friend.
- Others appreciate me and enjoy my company.

Fear of Making Mistakes

- I am sure of myself and my abilities.
- I am a quick thinker with an excellent memory.
- I accomplish what I set out to do effectively and correctly.

Fear of the Water

- I enjoy the feel of the water.
- I am an excellent swimmer.
- I can picture myself swimming with ease and confidence.

Fear of Specialization (you fill in the blanks)

- My ability to concentrate on one task is better than ever.
- I can picture myself being a _____, doing _____.
- I am more eager and enthusiastic than ever before to accomplish _____.

Fear of the Unknown

- I enjoy the challenge of exploring unfamiliar areas.
- I am totally calm and secure when I get lost.
- I like the adventure of new experiences.

Fear of Flying

- I am relaxed and at ease when I fly in a plane.
- I enjoy the peace and tranquility of flying high above the earth's surface.
- I have total trust in the pilot to fly the plane safely.

Fear of Taking Tests

- I become relaxed and confident when I enter a classroom to take a test.
- I read each question and problem with total understanding.
- My memory is clear with all the correct names, dates, places, concepts, and procedures.

Fear of Dying

- I have lived a full life and am calm and serene about taking the next step.
- I can leave this earth confident that I have made a valuable contribution to the lives of others.
- I am secure in knowing that I have made my peace with those who are important to me.

Fear of Making Decisions

- I am confident in my ability to make good decisions.
- I trust my judgment after considering both sides of an issue.
- I am more secure and self-assured than ever before about making choices that are correct for me and those around me.

Fear of Showing Your Feelings

- I am proud of who I am and look forward to sharing myself with others.
- I am secure about exposing my real self because I know that others will like me more for being open and honest.
- I am calm and self confident because I know I am responsible for my own emotions.

Fear of Not Having Enough Money

- I enjoy working and earning as much money as I need.
- I am confident that I can save 15% of every dollar that I earn.
- I can picture my savings account with a balance large enough for any emergency.

Fear of Going to the Dentist (Doctor)

- I have total confidence in my dentist (doctor) because I know he (she) will help me get better.
- I am calm, secure, and relaxed when I walk into the dentist's (doctor's) office.
- I am happy to see the dentist (doctor) because I know he (she) is kind, gentle, and considerate.

Fear of Change

- I look forward with enthusiasm to the new products and services that will become available next year.
- The more things change, the more relaxed I become because new things make my life easier.
- I get excited when I see things change because that creates opportunities for me to do what I'd like to do.

Fear of Animals or Spiders or Snakes

- I enjoy watching the behavior of animals as they go about their business.
- I am confident that insects and animals will respect my space so long as I respect theirs.
- I feel safe and secure in being considerate of other living beings.

Fear of Being a Victim of a Violent Crime

- I feel physically secure because I expect other people to be kind and considerate to me.
- I feel happy, peaceful and safe because I truly like and trust other people.
- The more threatening a situation becomes, the more relaxed and confident I become that it will resolve peacefully.

❖

Let's take stock of where you are on your journey of finding and exploring a new path for yourself—a path that leads to a fuller, richer and happier life. You have a map (what you are doing here); you have your compass (who you are); and you have cleared away a significant portion of the clutter in your way. You have begun overcoming your fears and excuses for not taking control of your life. All you need to do now is get rid of any remaining obstructions that have resulted from living a life that is out of balance or <u>too complicated</u>.

The next chapters will walk you through the steps you need to take to balance and simplify your life. Once you have accomplished those tasks, then you will be ready to start your journey toward the kind of positive and joyful future that you want to live.

> "A man can fail many times,
> but he isn't a failure
> until he begins
> to blame others."
> —Ted Engstrom

Chapter 5

How to Detect Imbalances in Your Life

People who lead a happy, successful and fulfilled life exercise all of their faculties: body, mind, emotions and instincts. To insure that your activities include a good balance of interests in the physical, mental, social and spiritual Areas of Life and also the cultural area, this chapter is like a radar screen. It will display any dangerous imbalances that may be obstructing your road to a happy, healthy, wealthy and wise future.

The steps in this chapter will help you uncover any tendencies you have to distort the natural balance of your life. Here you will

- Make a list of how you spend your time and classify these activities into the five Areas of Life. This will help you see if you are leading a life balanced among the five areas.

- Estimate on KEEPER #4—MY (AREA OF LIFE) ACTIVITIES how much time you spend on each activity. This will show you if the unbalanced use of your time is contributing to your stress, frustration and dissatisfaction in life.

- Record on KEEPER #5—MY WHEEL OF BALANCE, the percentage of time you spend on activities for each Area of Life. This will help you see if some of your faculties have atrophied to the point of powerlessness while others have become exhausted from overuse.

HOT TIP

> # Although you can't control the length of your life, you do have something to say about its width and depth.

Detecting your imbalances will be an eye-popping experience—a wake-up call that *you need to make some changes*. It is also an opportunity to make some logical improvements in your life. That realization should generate some self-confidence and give you hope for the future.

You have reached this chapter knowing your personal answers to questions many people never bother asking themselves:

- you understand who you are,

- you know why you are here, and

- you are either fearless or have begun the process of overcoming your fears.

But you didn't land in this chapter by mistake. The Self-Tests that you took back in the first chapter show that your life has more than its share of complications or imbalances. Each complication and imbalance is a personal obstruction, stopping you from moving along the road you want to travel. Together they are stopping you from making the important changes that will bring happiness, health, wealth and wisdom to you in the future.

When Your Life is Balanced, You Feel "Together"

You have already developed at least one Mission Statement for each of the five Areas of Life: Physical, Mental, Social, Spiritual and Cultural. No doubt you saw that although you devote most of your time and energy to roles in the cultural area, all five areas contain opportunities for your fulfillment. By paying attention to all five areas you bring balance to your life.

If you pay a visit to your local bookstore, you can find shelves of books about healthy living and philosophies of life. Most of them would tell you that BALANCE is essential. Everyone from Benjamin Franklin to Bertrand Russell, historian Arnold Toynbee, and scientist Jonas Salk agrees that when your life is out of balance, trouble begins.

You can nurture your complete well-being in four ways—each corresponding to an Area of Life. You can enrich your body by exercise and a good diet (Physical). You can nurture your mental self when you're studying a book or taking an adult education class on geography or government or whatever interests you (Mental). And when you are out socializing with people—whether you're dancing, talking, laughing or playing—you're giving your emotions a workout (Social). You develop your instincts when you have spiritual experiences such as communing with nature, meditating or attending a house of worship (Spiritual). These four Areas of Life—Physical, Mental, Social and Spiritual—provide you with the opportunity to nurture each of your four "natural" human gifts:

1. body,

2. mind,

3. emotions, and

4. instincts.

The Cultural area, on the other hand, provides you with diversions and allows you to develop your "marketable skills"— very tempting ways to spend your time. That's because there are strong forces at work in our society encouraging you to exercise these skills. Why? So you can earn a living, support a family, contribute to the economy and be a good citizen—all of which are good things to do and be.

Still, as important as the cultural area of life is, you should not neglect the growth and development of your body, mind, emotions, and instincts. These faculties are far more basic to your existence. Neglecting them will jack up your stress level, sap your energy, cloud your judgment and throw off your ability to understand clearly both yourself and the world around you. Allowing any of your fundamental "gifts" to atrophy will leave you wide open to becoming ill in one way or another.

An unbalanced life is like trying to walk proudly when one of your legs is shorter than the other. You can imagine how frustrating that would be. After a short time, your back would begin to hurt, both legs ache, your stride shorten as you hobble along. The imbalance would slow you down, keeping you from making the progress you want. And if you weren't careful, you would lose what balance you have and fall to the floor—probably ending up in a very embarrassing position!

A life that develops only one or two of the Areas of Life, while neglecting the others, is as out of balance as trying to walk with one leg shorter than the other. If you don't give full attention to all five Areas of Life, then you <u>are</u> in essence walking with one short leg, hindering yourself needlessly.

The results: Your life, just like your body, can fall down, plunging you into severe distress and unhappiness. You need to nurture each area of your life to lead a healthy existence.

My former boss in the corporate world is one of the prime examples I've personally observed. It shows what happens to someone who becomes preoccupied with the cultural area of life. He climbed up the corporate ladder so fast that he fell in love with his cultural standing, his power, and his money.

"Jim" became a vice president at the age of 35. He was addicted to his role—he didn't think he could live without it or that life outside of it was worth living. So his life began to revolve around making money, putting deals together and very little else. Jim was absorbed in the corporate life he was living. His level of stress mounted, but that stress acted as a kind of electricity keeping his motor running and his wheels turning. The corporate experience energized him, and he loved how he felt and what he could accomplish.

But only for a while. As his addiction grew, he put what little spiritual life he had on the shelf. That had never been particularly important to him anyway. He wasn't very athletic, so he postponed and finally neglected almost every bit of physical exercise. The only true exercise he had was sprinting between airline terminal gates to catch connecting flights.

For him, this lifestyle made sense. He believed that every hour of his time was too valuable. It was measured by the dollars he generated for himself and others. He was like H.L. Hunt, the Texas oil tycoon, who had a lifelong love of smoking cigars. Then he calculated that smoking each cigar consumed $6,000 worth of his time. As a multibillionaire, he could well afford the money by most any standard except his own. He decided that it wasn't worth the money to get a little pleasure out of life, so he gave up smoking cigars altogether.

My boss didn't smoke cigars, but he did give up anything he enjoyed that didn't relate to his job. He surrendered his intellectual interests outside the company. Instead, he exclusively read articles and memos concerning industry issues and corporate policies. When his wife divorced him, Jim simply picked a woman from within the organization to marry. By this time he was so addicted to his corporate role that he treated his new wife just like he would treat any other employee: He would give her orders and she was expected to follow them. By then, it was the only way he knew how to relate to people.

My former boss did nothing but live in the cultural area of life. In essence, by allowing himself to neglect the four natural Areas of Life in favor of the manmade cultural area, he was standing on one leg. And he was ready to fall.

It happened within a year after I left the company. His corporate accomplishments and roles started to bore him. He lost his zeal for making deals. The stress began to build to an unhealthy level. He wanted to control every person and situation he encountered, a need which drained his energy more, and more, and more. After a while, he just burned out. He was exhausted and drained. Jim reached a point where he just didn't care about work anymore, or anything else for that matter.

Because he had neglected the other four areas of life for so long, his natural support system had all but vanished. He had no friends outside the company. His body was flabby. He had no spiritual foundation to draw upon. He had lost perspective about what is important in life. His emphasis on money, material wealth, power, and control over others had drained him for so long he became a shell of a man before the age of 40. As a result, he lost his job, his wife, his power, his money and his self-respect. He fell far and long, paying a terrible price for living a life of IMBALANCE.

This example happens to be someone who overemphasized the cultural area of life. Although this affliction is definitely the most common type of imbalance you'll see, it is hardly the only one. No doubt you can think of examples of people you know, perhaps people very close to you, who became stuck in one Area of Life. Think of people you know as you read over this list of possibilities:

- people who are stuck in the social arena; They spend so much time with family and friends that they neglect to develop their minds and marketable skills.

- people who are stuck in the mental area; They go to school endlessly without ever <u>doing</u> anything with their lives.

- people who become consumed by spirituality to the point of religious fanaticism while ignoring opportunities for fulfillment in the other Areas of Life.

People who live such lopsided lives for any length of time find they can't keep it up. It's unhealthy! If they don't change their priorities consciously, then their body, mind, emotions, or instincts will force them to change. Burnout will be their wake-up call just like it was for my former boss. (Unfortunately, I lost track of him and don't know if he ever turned his life around.)

People who achieve happiness, and whatever else they want, live a balanced life in which they nurture and experience growth in all Areas of Life. Only then can they take advantage of the many, many opportunities for fulfillment that life offers. Only then can they develop and live up to their full potential. Only then can they effectively play principled roles that contribute to the lives of others while being a natural expression of who they really are.

> "The foolish man seeks happiness in the distance, the wise man grows it under his feet."
> —James Oppenheim

Are you ready to ensure that your life is balanced? Are you ready to make some changes that will not only simplify your existence but also create balance? If so, you are about to embark on a step-by-step journey that will help you remove the imbalances from your life and dispose of them permanently.

"How Do I Know When My Life Is Balanced?"

When your life is in balance, you experience feelings of inner peace. You know that you are spending your time correctly. You can focus on your activities with total concentration and commitment without nagging distractions from your subconscious. When you are trying to cope with an imbalance, you have twinges of uneasiness about what you are doing. These feelings manifest themselves as impatience and irritability showing the stress you're experiencing as you try to understand and deal with being "out of sync."

A useful tool to help you determine the degree of balance or imbalance in your life is the Wheel of Balance. It is a pictorial display of the five Areas of Life. Each area—cultural, mental, physical, social, and spiritual—represents a spoke of the wheel.

THE "IDEAL" WHEEL OF BALANCE

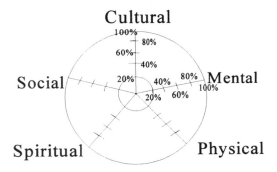

The Wheel of Balance illustrates the percentage of time spent on each of the Areas of Life.

Notice the crosshatches on each spoke. These lines each represent 20% of your time. Because there are five spokes, a perfectly balanced wheel will have a mark on the 20% crosshatch of each spoke for a total of 100%. The inner circle of the above "Ideal" wheel shows what your Wheel of Balance will look like if it is balanced: a perfect circular hub intersecting the 20% crosshatch for each spoke. This is an ideal which should be your target, your long-range goal.

Leading a balanced life does not mean that every 60 minutes must be divided into five equal (12-minute) intervals giving equal time to each area every hour. Similarly, if you sleep for nine hours, leaving 15 waking hours, you don't have to spend three hours each day on each Area of Life to achieve daily balance. Nor does it mean that during a 30-day month you need to spend exactly six days on each Area of Life each day.

Life is to be lived, not calibrated down to the minute by apportioning your time according to some rigid system. But in the long run, you need to be devoting approximately 20% of your time to each area, on the average, to lead a balanced life.

You know what happens to an automobile tire which isn't weighted properly all the way around. It wobbles. The tire wears out. The front end shimmies. The car becomes difficult to steer and you can lose control. A little imbalance in your automobile tire can cause you a lot of stress, cost you a lot of money and become a big safety hazard.

The same is true of your life's Wheel of Balance. If one or more of the areas of your life are not weighted properly, your life becomes lopsided and you are in danger of losing control. You must fix that situation before you jeopardize your future health, wealth, wisdom, and happiness.

Step 1: How Do You Spend Your Time?

When you stop and think about it, what's the one resource we all have in common? That's right, TIME! We all have time but we sure don't use it in the same way. There are so many activities to choose from that no two people use their time in exactly the same way. The trouble with time is that once you've spent it, it's gone! There's no refund. You can't get it back.

There are no second chances. You can't spend your time in the past any differently. You can, however, make a conscious effort to allocate your time wisely in the future.

To live a life of success, happiness and fulfillment, you need to lead a balanced life. You need to allocate your time to the five areas of life. When you do that, your Wheel of Balance approaches a nice round hub in the center intersecting the 20% crosshatch on each of those spokes in the long run. Otherwise, you will be harboring imbalances, frittering away your time and delaying your opportunity for a life of fulfillment.

So, let's see how you are spending your time. MY ACTIVITIES WORKSHEET will get you started. You need to list all of the activities that consume your time. If you draw a blank, turn to KEEPER #1—MY RESOURCES that you have already completed in the KEEPER Forms Section. Remind yourself of "The Activities I Enjoy Most."

These activities certainly don't include all of the ways you spend you time. To help you come up with some additional ways, here's a reprint of the "Interests" section of Table I. These are sample activities for each Area of Life.

(INTERESTS)

CULTURAL	MENTAL	PHYSICAL	SOCIAL	SPIRITUAL
Watch TV	Read	Work out	Date	Meditate
Go school	Do Xword	Walk	Gatherings	Go to church
Go to movie	Take notes	Compete	Parties	Go on retreat
Housework	Study	Dance	"Hang out"	See nature
Drive car	Do research	Groom	Socials	Pray
Go to work	Surf "net"		"Do lunch"	Heal self
Buy things	Watch PBS			Keep diary

When listing activities, be sure to distinguish between the various Areas of Life. "Going to school," for example, is a cultural activity. "Studying" is a mental activity. Similarly, "Working out in the gym" is a physical activity but "driving to and from the gym" is a cultural experience. In fact all the driving you do is cultural in nature and should be listed separately from the activities themselves: "driving to/from work," "driving to/from school," "driving to/from the gym," "driving to/from church," etc.

You will tend to associate most activities with only one of the five Areas of Life. For example, "shopping" is clearly cultural. "Worshiping in church" is clearly spiritual. "Going to parties" is definitely social. But some activities may involve a strong secondary Area of Life as well.

To give you a personal example, I sing with a barbershop quartet. For me, this is primarily a spiritual experience. My instincts take over when I am singing and recreating the composer's message through the melody, harmony and lyrics of the piece. It doesn't matter how many times we sing a song, I always experience the spiritual effects.

Sometimes this intuitive sense is very strong. Sometimes it is weaker. But, it is always present whether we are practicing or performing. Secondary to all of this is the social aspect of interacting with the three other guys. It takes a real commitment and rapport with each other to prepare and maintain a 50-song repertoire.

If I had to approximate the allocation between these two Areas of Life, I would estimate that barbershop singing for me is 70% spiritual and 30% social. But, ask the other three guys and you would probably get entirely different answers.

This experience is very personal and individual. In fact, one of my barbershop quartet buddies might say that, for him, the mental area is more important. He enjoys using his mind to learn and memorize the words, notes, dynamics and gestures. Another of us four might consider the cultural aspect of performing or the physical aspect of producing the musical sounds to be the most important. For me, those considerations are minor.

The most important thing to do as you fill out MY ACTIVITIES WORKSHEET is to put each activity in the category or categories that fit for you. Try to limit yourself to the primary category unless a secondary one really seems significant. Only on the most time-consuming activities, such as your job, should you ever consider a third category.

Remember, this list is just an approximation. There are no penalties for being "off" by 10%, 20% or even 30%. Whatever you list on MY ACTIVITIES WORKSHEET will put you on track for determining which of your faculties are overworked and which are underused. Only after you identify the nature of your imbalances can you take corrective action to gain control of your life.

Here are the entries on MY ACTIVITIES WORKSHEET completed by "Betty" one of my workshop participants. Review her entries. Then make your own list of all the activities on which you spend time using MY ACTIVITIES WORKSHEET on the subsequent page.

"The reward
of a thing well done
is
to have done it well."

—Ralph Waldo Emerson

MY ACTIVITIES WORKSHEET (Sample for "Betty")

How I Spend My Time	Physical	Mental	Social	Spirit	Cultural
Administrative Job		20%	20%		60%
Travel to Job					100%
Study		100%			
Attend Church				100%	
Travel to Church					100%
Workout at Gym	80%		20%		
Travel to Gym					100%
Read Novels		100%			
Do Crossword Puzzles		100%			
Do House/Yard Work	50%				50%
Go to Parties			100%		
Travel to Parties					100%
Watch TV					100%
Watch PBS-TV		100%			
Go Shopping					100%
Travel to Shop					100%
Eat Alone	100%				
Eat with Others	50%		50%		
Groom	50%				50%
Meditate				100%	
Attend Club Meetings					100%
Research on Internet		100%			
Keep a Diary				100%	
Walk Somewhere	80%			20%	

MY ACTIVITIES WORKSHEET

How I Spend My Time	Physical	Mental	Social	Spirit	Cultural

"On the road to success,
you're not just learning from
your own experiences."
—Rick Patino

Step 2: But Do You Know HOW MUCH Time You Spend?

So, now you can see in black and white how you spend your time, what Area of Life you favor and which you tend to neglect. But, to see the actual MAGNITUDE of the imbalances you're living with, you need to do some calculating. Yeah, I know you haven't used your calculator for a while. But this is easy stuff and the payoff is big. You'll observe firsthand how your unbalanced use of time is contributing to the stress, frustration and dissatisfaction in your life.

You need to figure out approximately how many hours you devote to each Area of Life in a typical year. That's right, a year. Why? Because imbalances can be tolerated for a couple of weeks or even months because of life's necessities, or even for sheer pleasure. A year gives you a more realistic perspective of how you generally spend your time. These calculations will involve estimating how much time you spend on each activity that you have just listed on MY ACTIVITIES WORKSHEET.

There is room for you to do these calculations on KEEPER

#4—MY (AREA OF LIFE) ACTIVITIES. As with your other important documents, there is a KEEPER #4 in the KEEPER Forms Section for each Area of Life. For starters, you need to transcribe the activities from MY ACTIVITIES WORKSHEET on to the appropriate Area of Life form. For example, referring to Betty's ACTIVITIES WORKSHEET, she created a KEEPER #4—MY PHYSICAL ACTIVITIES containing the following entries: workout at gym, do house/yard work, eat alone, eat with others, groom and walk somewhere.

KEEPER #4 is particularly important because you will be using it not only here but also when you develop ideas for simplifying and balancing your life. Right now, you will only be working with the left-hand side—your "Current Activities."

The right-hand side of KEEPER #4, your "Ideas for Change," will come into play in the next chapter. There you will record the beginnings of a plan to simplify your life and bring it into better balance. You will be amazed at the results. They will be dramatic!

On page 168 you will find Betty's completed KEEPER #4—MY CULTURAL ACTIVITIES based on her worksheet.

The first cultural activity from her ACTIVITIES WORKSHEET is her administrative job. The 60% figure was her own estimate of how much of the time she spent on the job actually involved the use of her marketable administrative skills, rather than socializing (20%) or reading (20%).

The calculation here is 40 hours per week times 50 weeks (she gets a two-week vacation) equaling 2000 hours at 60% or <u>1200 hours.</u> This information is recorded as the first "Current Activity" on her KEEPER #4—MY CULTURAL ACTIVITIES.

Driving your car is primarily a cultural activity. Why? For the most part, you're not exercising your body, mind, emotions or intuition when you are driving. You're pretty much on "cruise control," doing little except keeping the car on the road and out of crashes. Some people—chauffeurs, cab drivers, bus and truck drivers get paid for driving. They're probably exercising a lot more skill than you or I might, however, and that's why for them driving is a marketable commodity.

My workshop participant drove to several of her activities, and here's how she broke down the time she spent:

- work (30 minutes each way) took her five hours per week and 250 hours per year—no commuting during her two weeks vacation (5 hrs/week * 50 weeks = 250 hours).

- church (15 minutes each way) took her 30 minutes per week for 50 weeks a year or 25 hours per year.

- the gym which she frequented twice a week was also 15 minutes from home (1/2 hour * 2 times/wk * 50 weeks = 50 hours per year).

- the weekly parties she attended also involved an average of 30 minutes of driving (30 minutes * 50 weeks = 25 hours per year).

These driving times were added up and entered as "Current Activity" #2 on MY CULTURAL ACTIVITIES.

Table III

"Betty's" Driving Times

DRIVING ACTIVITY	HOURS
Work	250
Church	25
Gym	50
Parties	25
GRAND TOTAL	350 hours

The third "Current Activity," doing housework took Betty an average of two hours per week which equates to 100 hours each and every year.

Watching network TV is her fourth "Current Activity." Spending only two hours a day in front of the "telly" consumed an astonishing 700 HOURS PER YEAR. Here's the calculation: 2 hrs per day * 7 days/wk * 50 weeks = 700 hours/year.

Shopping and running errands is a common cultural activity. Betty did three hours worth every week (including the driving time to and from the shops). Excluding her vacationing, that's 3 hrs/wk * 50 wks = 150 hours per year.

Her sixth cultural activity involved a club she belonged to. Each week she attended this group's meeting which lasted an average of two hours. That involvement added another (2 hrs/wk * 50wks =) 100 hours to her annual consumption of cultural hours.

MY CULTURAL ACTIVITIES

Current	Ideas for Change
1. Work at admin job: 40 hrs * 50 wks * 60% = <u>1200</u> hrs	1. _____hrs
2. Drive car: 250+25+50+25 = <u>350</u> hrs	2. _____hrs
3. Do house/yard work: 2 hrs * 50 wks = <u>100</u> hrs	3. _____hrs
4. Watch network TV 2 hrs * 7 days * 50 wks = <u>700</u> hrs	4. _____hrs
5. Shop/run errands 3 hrs * 50 wks = <u>150</u> hrs	5. _____hrs
6. Attend club meeting 2 hrs * 50 wks = <u>100</u> hrs	6. _____hrs
7. _____hrs	7. _____hrs
8. _____hrs	8. _____hrs

TOTAL HOURS ____2600____   TOTAL HOURS_____

% CULTURAL ____44.6%____   % CULTURAL _____

Now that the individual estimates have been recorded, let's see how much time Betty accumulated for all of the activities in her Cultural Area of Life:

ACTIVITY	TIME
Work	1200
Driving	350
House/Yard Work	100
Network TV	700
Shop/Run Errands	150
Club Meetings	100
GRAND TOTAL	2600 Hours

That's a total of 2,600 hours per year that she was spending exercising her marketable skills and cultural diversions. Sure, that seems like a lot of hours, but let's see how it measures up on a percentage basis.

Most people sleep an average eight hours a night. That means you are awake and able to devote time to Areas of Life activities an average of 16 hours each day. This equates to about 5824 HOURS PER YEAR! (That's 16 times 364 days per year.)

Result: Betty's 2,600 hours of "cultural time" corresponds to 44.6% of the hours she had available. That's not the 20% ideal. It's not even close! Her cultural time was gobbling up almost half of her life. She was letting some of her basic faculties—body, mind, emotions and intuition—wither.

Have you fallen into a similar trap? Are you spending way too much time in one Area of Life while neglecting others? There's an easy way to check. Make the calculations as Betty did. *You be the judge*. The evidence will be right there in front of you.

Remember, the 20% target for each Area of Life is just that—something to shoot for over the course of a lifetime. Depending on your age, circumstances may require you to emphasize one of the areas more than the others.

For example, if you're still completing your education, you probably are spending more than 20% of your time in the mental Area of Life. During mid-life most people devote extra time to the cultural area because they have become established in a career and are finishing the task of raising children. Once retirement comes into play, people often focus more on their spirituality as they contemplate their own mortality.

So, you need to decide for yourself how to modify the 20% long-term averages at your particular stage of life. Don't try to kid yourself, though. You can only get away with temporary imbalances for short periods. If you continue to over-exercise your marketable skills in the cultural area while your basic human faculties (body, mind, emotions and instincts) are allowed to shrivel, you'll meet the same brick wall as my ex-boss—BURNOUT.

Let's finish this step in the process of identifying the imbalances in your life. Figure out the percentage of time you give to each Area of Life using KEEPER #4 found in the KEEPER Forms Section. Do the calculations in small steps just as Betty did for KEEPER #4—MY CULTURAL ACTIVITIES. On KEEPER #4, record your estimate of how many hours per year you spend on each of your activities. Calculate your estimates using the same methods she did. To figure out how much time you spend on each area, add up the number of hours for each activity in that area.

When you add up the totals for each area, you should get a grand total that corresponds to your total number of waking hours in the year. Table IV shows you how the number of hours you are awake in a year corresponds to the "average hours of sleep" you get each night.

Table IV

AVERAGE HOURS OF SLEEP	NUMBER OF HOURS AWAKE
(per night)	(per year)
5	6912
6	6552
7	6188
8	5824
9	5460
10	5096

If the grand total of the hours you spend on your activities doesn't match the number of hours you are awake in a year, you have some fine-tuning to do. Perhaps you left out some activities or maybe you didn't estimate your times properly. Either way, you need to go back and juggle the numbers until the two totals come within a couple hundred hours of each other. That's close enough for the purpose of identifying the major imbalances in your life.

Step 3: Are You Leading a Balanced Life?

You've just done some serious calculating. As you take one final step, you will uncover the percentage of time you're spending on each area. You will be able to see on KEEPER #5—MY BALANCE WHEEL which of your faculties have begun to atrophy and which are suffering from overuse.

Divide the hours spent in each area by your total waking hours per year and then multiply by 100. Presto! You have the percentage of time you are currently spending in each Area of Life. This is what "Betty" did to calculate the 44.6% for her cultural activities:

$$\frac{\text{Cultural hours}}{\text{Waking hours}} = \frac{2600}{5824} = .446 \times 100 = 44.6\%$$

After making these calculations, record your results on the bottom of KEEPER #4—MY (AREA OF LIFE) ACTIVITIES and on the following chart under the heading "THE ACTUAL YOU."

YOUR ALLOCATION OF TIME

Area of Life	The Ideal "You"	The Actual "You"	The Practical "You"
Cultural	20%	%	%
Mental	20%	%	%
Physical	20%	%	%
Social	20%	%	%
Spiritual	20%	%	%
TOTALS	100%	100%	100%

So, what's the verdict? Do you allocate your time in a balanced fashion? How close do you come to those 20% targets for each area? Considering that you are concentrating on this Chapter, achieving balance must be a problem for you. I'm guessing your figures show that you have some large variations from the ideal.

If you feel that the "Ideal" targets of 20% are impractical for you because of your age, make your own targets in the third Column—The Practical You. If you are tempted to increase an Area of Life above the 20% Ideal, remember that your faculties get tired just like you do. What happens when you're overtired? You don't function properly. Same thing happens when your body, mind, emotions or instincts are overused. They don't work right!

When one Area of Life is increased, others must be decreased below the 20% Ideal. Using one of your faculties to a lesser amount is unhealthy because you won't exercise it enough.

What happens if your arm has to be in a cast? The muscles atrophy and don't work right. The same thing can happen to your mind, emotions, instincts or marketable skills. If you don't use them, you lose them. So, be very careful about establishing Practical percent allocations that differ significantly from the 20% Ideal for any length of time. Live happily, healthfully & wisely—live a balanced life.

To complete the snapshot of your current life, put your Actual percentage allocations of time on the appropriate crosshatches of KEEPER #5—MY WHEEL OF BALANCE. Each crosshatch is 10% greater than the previous one. So, if one of your allocations is 15%, you should place it halfway between the crosshatches representing 10% and 20%. You've got the idea!

After marking all five of your points on the Wheel of Balance, go ahead and "connect the dots." Remember that the ideal allocation results in a perfectly round circular hub on the Wheel of Balance.

MY WHEEL OF BALANCE

Percentage of Time Spent in Each Area of Life

(Before Changes)

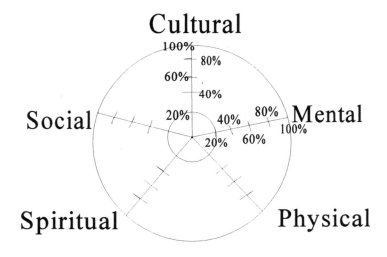

What does your allocation look like? How would you like to be riding on a wheel as unbalanced as that? I think you've got some repair work to do before you get back on the road. Are you ready to do what it takes to introduce some balance into your life? If so, you're ready to start simplifying! Making moves to simplify your life is the next step toward creating a balanced life. At the same time, simplification will clear away any clutter in your life and provide the <u>time and space</u> you need to make some positive changes for your future. How can you pass up an opportunity like that?

Take a deep breath. You've just about finished a road map of how you spend your time now. In the next chapter, I will show you how you can "buy some time" in the future by making changes that will simplify your life <u>and</u> eliminate some of your imbalances. However, you must be willing to make changes. You must be willing to discard old habits which are now standing in the way of the kind of life you want and deserve.

> "We make our habits
> and then
> our habits make us."
> —Stephen Covey

PAYOFF BOX

I spend too much time doing _____ _____.
For the next week I will spend 30 minutes less each day on that activity. In its place I will do something in the Area of Life where I spend the least amount of time. At the end of the week, I will reflect on the increased satisfaction I have experienced.

Chapter 6

How to Create Balance
by
Simplifying Your Life

People who are happy, healthy and fulfilled enjoy simple lives. They avoid the complexities that cause worry, stress, disease and unhealthful lifestyles. "Simple" doesn't mean they live a life so elementary that they inhabit thatched huts and gather berries. It means their lives are uncluttered purposely, free from distractions which serve only to complicate, not enrich their lives.

Right now, you have a terrific chance to get the obstacles complicating your life out of your pathway. You can simplify your life and make it far better than it has been.

You've already identified the Areas of Life where you are spending far too much time. This chapter will get you going on the step-by-step process of bringing your life into better balance. How? By giving your overused faculties a stress-reducing break. Here's what you'll do:

- You'll review some guidelines for deciding how to simplify your life and prepare your subconscious to help you with the process. Result: You'll free up precious time to make the positive changes you need to make.

- You'll record your Ideas for Change on KEEPER #4—MY (AREA OF LIFE) ACTIVITIES. Here, you'll determine the amount of time you will save and the amount of time you will spend on each AREA OF LIFE in the future. Result: You will experience bone-deep satisfaction as you lift a huge weight off your shoulders. You'll also have much more self-respect as you start doing only the things that *really* matter to you.

You began working with KEEPER #4 when you were detecting the imbalances in your life. Now you will complete these important milestones to simplify your life while creating a balanced lifestyle. Here's your opportunity to share two more characteristics with happy people: living balanced and living simply.

> "In order to grow,
> you must give something up.
> You must abandon
> the unproductive and
> worthless to free up resources
> for other things."
> —Peter Drucker

When Your Life is Simple, You Feel "in control"

Let's cut right to the chase. Complexities in life cause stress. Although some stress is good for you, too much stress causes ill health. Ill health, in turn, causes premature death. The antidote for this downward spiral is simplicity. Simplicity in life lowers your stress level, nourishes good health and lets you live longer. It's that simple!

Well, no, not really. Like most of life, it's more complicated than that. Changes are happening all around you, and you have no control over many of them. Though you may have no control over them, they certainly can have an impact on you. Some changes, like advances in modern technology, tend to make life easier for you. Others, like bureaucracy, add a level of complexity that your ancestors did not have to deal with which often brings unnecessary stress and complications.

For example, the modern portable phone with such features as touch-tone dialing, memory buttons, and automatic redial, genuinely saves you time and adds convenience to your life. It's a big improvement over the old stationary, rotary dial phones.

However, your ancestors are probably spinning in their crypts over the complicated income tax laws that now require you to pay more to have your tax return prepared than they ever had to pay in taxes.

Even with all the modern conveniences that add genuine benefit to your life, getting snared in all the demands of modern society is far too easy. For example, roads and highways are better and cars are safer and more comfortable than they were. Unfortunately, most people find themselves driving farther and more often than was necessary in previous generations.

Television reception is greatly improved since its inception. You have many, many program choices. The remote control that came with your TV will do everything except pop your corn.

However, the temptation to watch TV becomes more and more compelling. Why? You're wiped out! Your job and your family, if you have one, squeeze so much out of you that you haven't the time or energy left over to go out for quality entertainment. This cultural drain on your time, energy, and attention can, and usually does, complicate your life without enriching it.

Don't blame it all on technology, though. That's too easy. People do their share of the damage, too. Some will push you as far as you let them. That includes even the most well-meaning and considerate of your friends and relatives, your spouse or significant other, and your children.

They all want to know if you can help them with "this or that." They want to know if you want to go "here or there." They ask if you have any of "these or those" that they can borrow or keep. Their demands can gobble up valuable time and energy.

Then there's your job. Earning a living probably eats up more of your time, puts more demands on you and your resources, than any other pressure. Most people have to work at least 40 hours a week during 50 weeks a year. In this era of downsizing and operating lean and mean, jobs can require much more time than the standard 40-hour work week.

All of these demands and pressures come crashing down on you like a rock slide on your road to happiness; they can easily overwhelm and control you. The result? Stress, ill health, shorter life. (Remember?)

You need to get out from under that rock slide. You need to move away from that disaster. You need to get on the road you want to travel after removing the debris that is getting in your way.

A main purpose of this chapter is to clear away that clutter by simplifying your life. You need to find some breathing room. You need some space that will allow you to kick those obstacles to the side of the road and redirect the future course of your life. That way you can travel the road <u>you</u> want to travel.

Just believing in simplicity is not enough; you have to stitch it into the fiber of your being. If you want to lead a happy, stress-free, healthy and long life, first you have to start talking about simplicity, then put it into motion.

RESOURCE BOX

The "father" of contemporary views on simplicity is Duane Elgin, who wrote his landmark book called <u>Voluntary Simplicity</u> in 1979. He is a strong advocate of such principles as respect for the earth, frugality and spiritual fulfillment.

Step 1: Some Guidelines to Help You Find Simplicity

As you begin the task of simplifying your life, here are some tips to guide your thinking. These hints will enable you to adjust your activities while improving the complete quality of your life.

1   Trim back activities which have become routine and even boring. They already have served their purpose both as growth experiences and as stabilizing influences in your life. Now may be the time to let go of them and make room for something more fulfilling in the future. *That's what happened to me when I gave up my yard work and hired it out. A balanced life needs to contain new interests as well as old standbys.* So, when you take a look at your KEEPER #4—MY (AREA OF LIFE) ACTIVITIES, see if you can spot some things you'd like to modify. You may even dump some things that you don't really enjoy anymore.

2   Cut out interests that seem to drain you and leave you feeling empty. Instead, look for activities that energize you. Otherwise, you'll just fritter away time doing things which sap you, robbing you of opportunities for fulfillment. *For example, if battling morning and evening rush hour traffic leaves you feeling dragged out, give the alternatives some* _real_ *consideration. Maybe you'll find reading on public transit or riding in an amiable carpool a real energizer.* As you review MY (AREA OF LIFE) ACTIVITIES, dig deep for the courage to reduce or eliminate things you're doing that are only marginally useful, or perhaps harmful.

3   If your schedule is loaded with activities in which you have to be in control, give some serious thought to balancing things out with some interests where you can just "hang out." *For example, if you're a leader in your PTA or business organization, think about joining another organization where you don't have to lead.* A balanced life should contain a mix of situations: some in which you call the shots, and some in which you follow the lead of others. Look over your activities closely with this control feature in mind.

4   Stress can be a motivator—up to a point. But if one or more of your activities has reached the point of DIS-stress, give a little <u>extra</u> consideration to ways of reducing or eliminating them. *For example, if shopping really gets on your nerves and causes you to have physical problems, <u>it ain't good for you</u> and you know it. Figure out a way to do it less; maybe you could even get someone else to do it for you in exchange for your doing something for them.* A balanced life contains a manageable amount of stress. Life is too short to tolerate stresses that make it even shorter. You need to think about stress while you look over your activities during this simplification process. Too much stress will damage your mind, your body, your emotions and your intuition. Preserve them all. Cut down on your stress.

5   A balanced life is one in which you help some people and allow others to help you. If your current activities tip this scale too far in one direction or the other, you need to reduce or eliminate a few of those. *As you consider the entries on MY*

(AREA OF LIFE) ACTIVITIES, see if you are overly committed to helping others. You know you can't be all things to all people. It's exhausting and impossible. Trying to be what everyone wants you to be will only stretch you to the breaking point. You may need to practice saying "no" a bit more often. You're the only one who can come up with some simpler alternatives that will provide you with some much-needed breathing room. The expression "Just say no" applies to more than drugs. It also applies to you and your life if your life is too unbalanced or too complicated for you to take control of your own future.

> "OPPORTUNITIES never come
> to those who wait.....
> they are captured by those
> who dare to ATTACK."
> —Paul J. Meyer

I know you are convinced that simplifying your life is the best thing to do. It will reduce your level of stress. It will improve your health. You will have time to make improvements in your life. And, it will increase your longevity. But this understanding is only on a conscious level.

You must dig deeper. Is your subconscious going to accept all this? Will your subconscious let you prune away some interests and activities that may have grown into being as much a part of your life as some longtime buddies you've outgrown? Some relationships are bad habits. Better assume that your subconscious needs more prodding before you start getting some unnecessary resistance.

To help you break down any resistance, memorize the following affirmation: I AM ANXIOUS TO SIMPLIFY MY LIFE SO I CAN USE THE TIME THAT I FREE UP TO CREATE A MORE FULFILLING FUTURE.

As with other messages intended for your subconscious, this affirmation needs to be repeated again and again in the days ahead. During your quiet time, repeat it five or six times in a row. Allow it to soak into your subconscious mind while you are in a relaxed and meditative state. Do it before you go to sleep at night and when you first awake in the morning. Both times are excellent opportunities to present this TRUTH to your subconscious. The result: Your subconscious will help you during the simplification tasks ahead.

Step 2: "Buying Time" by Simplifying Your Activities

One or more of your (AREA OF LIFE) ACTIVITIES will show a total of more than 20% of your time. These are the areas where you need to focus right now. You must concentrate on these areas to clear away the clutter. These areas contain your opportunities for simplification. The others, for now, are not as critical.

RESOURCE BOX

> One of the best treatments of our society's preoccupation with the Cultural Area of Life and the risks of not creating balance and simplicity has been written by Vicki Robin and Joe Dominguez—"Your Money or Your Life."

I have the feeling that your Cultural Area of Life exceeds 20%. So, to demonstrate the process of freeing up time by simplifying your activities, let's continue the example introduced in the last chapter. You remember Betty, one of my workshop participants. We examined the left side of her page—"Current Activities." Now let's see how she simplified her cultural activities.

There are only three ways to simplify an area of your life:

1   eliminate an activity completely;

2   reduce the total time you spend on an activity, or

3   convert an activity so that some or all of the time saved gets moved to another Area of Life.

Let's look at each one of Betty's cultural activities. First, we'll review how much time she currently spends on it. Then we'll consider some simplification ideas so it consumes less cultural time.

Because her job is close to her heart—it does pay the bills, after all—it required more attention than some of her other activities. She reported that her administrative job had expanded to the point where she was expected to be too many things for too many people.

Deadlines had overlapped and she found herself being pulled in too many directions at once. At the same time, she was becoming bored with many of her tasks because she had done them so often that they had become routine.

Betty was suffering from two occupational hazards, stress and apathy. Both are far too common in the workplace. Here are some ideas for change that she and I discussed:

- Job modification . . . hiring an assistant to perform some routine tasks allowing her to spend 20% of her time on strategic planning, where she can exercise her brain. This is an example of converting cultural time to mental time to alleviate both distress and boredom.

- Job sharing . . . arranging to share responsibilities with another person of comparable skills at the same level. Such an improvement would have the potential of reducing both stress and apathy. It would also convert some of her cultural time to social time that she could use to nurture the relationship with the person with whom she was sharing.

- Job change . . . looking for a job in this or another organization in which her role would be more compatible with her personality. This change should relieve stress and be an energizing move. It will also convert her current job mix of 20% mental, 20% social and 60% cultural, to some new percentage allocation which would be more balanced.

- Career change . . . training for a new career has the same potential benefits as a job change with the opportunity to consider many more alternatives.

Notice on the right-hand side of her KEEPER #4—MY CULTURAL ACTIVITIES (page 193) that Betty has recorded all four of these "Ideas for Change." However, she has underlined only the first one, Job modification. That's because she felt it was the most practical option and the one she wanted to adopt. She recalculated the cultural time she would be spending on her job using this job modification.

Hiring an assistant would convert 20% of her cultural time to mental time. The change would mean her new job mix would be 40% mental, 20% social and only 40% cultural. Consequently, her modified job would consume 40% of 40 hours times 50 weeks or 800 cultural hours per year.

As you recall, Betty also spent 350 cultural hours per year driving her car in connection with four separate activities. She decided that driving to work was the only part of this activity she wanted to consider simplifying. Commuting was particularly bothersome because fighting that traffic was a real drain on her energy. She would often arrive at work frazzled by the drive. Having to face the rush hour after a long day on the job was one of her least favorite things about working.

One idea she had for saving some of this cultural time was to carpool to work. By joining with four others, she would only have to drive 1/5th of the time. Instead of spending 250 hours annually driving to work, her commute driving would be reduced to only 50 hours per year (1/5th of 250).

As a passenger, she could convert those 200 hours of cultural time to mental time by reading or to social time by becoming friends with her fellow commuters. Maybe she could even sleep some of the time. In any case, she would substitute potentially energizing activities in other Areas of Life for the draining cultural activity, driving to and from work.

Besides carpooling, Betty considered public transportation as another "Idea for Change." She could read, sleep or socialize on public buses and trains. She could also meditate, to get in some spiritual time, if she wanted.

Are you starting to get the hang of how you can begin creating balance in your life? You must change some activities so you convert time spent in one Area of Life to another Area of Life.

Betty also considered reducing the time she spent commuting by moving closer to work. Although she had compelling reasons for living where she did, the prospect of SAVING 250 hours of precious time—and then converting it to some quality activities in areas where she wasn't spending enough time—made her think long and hard. What an opportunity!

Finally, though, she decided to choose the carpool alternative. You will notice that it is underlined on the right-hand side on her KEEPER #4—MY CULTURAL ACTIVITIES—and is the basis for reducing her driving hours from 350 to 150 per year.

The third cultural activity, doing housework, currently took her two hours per week or 100 hours annually. She'd been doing housework for many years, and it had become a boring and dull chore a long, long time ago.

When she realized she was spending 100 hours every year, she decided to hire someone to do it from then on. "Why do something I've grown to despise when I make good money and can pay to have it done for me?" she said.

You'll notice that there is only one "Idea for Change" for cultural activity number three because she made the decision to <u>Hire someone to do it</u>. Consequently, the hours spent here are now zero.

Consider this fundamental rule: THE BEST WAY to simplify your life is to completely eliminate doing something. Obviously, that's not always possible. Even so, it is the absolute best way.

As you look over the rest of Betty's cultural activities sheet, review how the process works. Basically, you let your subconscious help you come up with ways to cut down or eliminate the number of hours you currently spend doing something. In some cases you will come up with ideas for converting an activity to another Area of Life—preferably to one in which you are currently spending less than 20% of your time. Remember, pruning away activities which bore you, drain your energy, create an unhealthy imbalance or just plain stress you out is going to free up time that you can use to substitute something that energizes you.

For example, Betty was watching network TV for only two hours a day. When she calculated it was consuming 700 HOURS PER YEAR, she was stunned. That's more than 10% of the waking hours she had available! When your body, mind, emotions, or instincts are crying out for exercise, being a couch potato is a terrible way to use your time.

Betty needed to be more judicious about her network TV viewing. She had allowed herself to fall into the cultural habit of watching TV for a couple of hours each evening until it was time to go to bed. She even admitted that she was bored by most of the programs. NOT GOOD.

She came up with two "Ideas for Change" to fix this problem. First, Betty considered developing an interest in the more mentally stimulating PBS Television programs. Secondly, she tried to be more selective about her network TV habit. She decided to carefully choose four of her favorite shows <u>each week</u> to serve as her cultural diversion—two half-hour sitcoms and two one-hour series.

These changes would lower the number of hours she spent in front of "the tube" to 150 annually (3 hours per week times 50 weeks per year). That's a savings of 550 hours! Now we're talking about freeing up some serious time. How would you like "to be given 550 free hours" to use when you begin mapping out your future life of happiness and fulfillment?

Betty's fifth current cultural activity was shopping and running errands which consumed three hours per week. She considered doing this with a friend to convert some of the time to the Social Area of Life. But, she decided on a second "Idea for Change"—only doing it biweekly. She was quite sure that three hours would still be adequate. Consequently, she cut the time for this activity in half (3 hours times 25 times per year is 75 hours annually).

Her club meetings were a cultural experience where she had chosen to play a leadership role. Realizing she was playing a leadership role at work as well, she decided to rethink the situation. She saw that she could create more balance in her life if she were involved in something in which she was <u>not</u> in control. She considered eliminating the Club completely. Instead, she decided to become a social member rather than a leader. That meant her club meeting instantly became social time instead of cultural time.

By making the changes outlined on her example of the cultural activities sheet, Betty could reduce her annual allocation of cultural <u>hours</u> from 2,600 down to 1,175. Based on her total available hours of 5,824 annually (remember she slept an average of eight hours per night), she could slash to 20.2% the amount of time she spent exercising her marketable skills and cultural diversions. But she could do that only if she put into gear <u>all</u> of her selected "Ideas for Change." If she did, she would make a very significant step in the direction of <u>both</u> simplifying and balancing her life.

"We are confronted with insurmountable opportunities."

—Walt Kelley

MY CULTURAL ACTIVITIES

Current	Ideas for Change
1. Work at admin job: 40 hrs * 50 wks * 60% = 1200 hrs	1. Career change Job sharing or change Job modification 800 hrs
2. Drive car: 250+25+50+25 = 350 hrs	2. Take public transport Live closer to work Carpool to work 150 hrs
3. Do house/yard work: 2 hrs * 50 wks = 100 hrs	3. Hire someone to do it 0 hrs
4. Watch network TV 2 hrs * 7 days * 50 wks = 700 hrs	4. Develop PBS interest Be more selective 150 hrs
5. Shop/run errands 3 hrs * 50 wks = 150 hrs	5. Go with a friend Go biweekly 75 hrs
6. Attend club meeting 2 hrs * 50 wks = 100 hrs	6. Eliminate Join a different club Be social member 0 hrs
7. _____hrs	7. _____hrs
8. _____hrs	8. _____hrs

TOTAL HOURS ____2600____	TOTAL HOURS____1175____
% CULTURAL ____44.6%____	% CULTURAL ____20.2%____

Okay, spread out each of your sheets, KEEPER #4—MY (AREA OF LIFE) ACTIVITIES. Remember, these forms are perforated in the KEEPER Forms Section for easy removal and copying. Concentrate on the Areas of Life that show a current percentage time exceeding 20% and start pruning. As a reminder, here's how to liberate your subconscious and let it get to work on finding you some Ideas for Change. Just find a quiet place where you won't be interrupted for a while. Now <u>trust</u> your subconscious to identify some feasible alternatives.

As Betty did in the example, write down all the possibilities that come to mind even if you've rejected them in the past. Don't let any idea slip by, no matter how bizarre, impossible, dumb or uninteresting it may seem. You know what happens to a bottle of soda after you shake it up. It gets all fizzy and starts spurting out of the bottle. That's what you want to do here. Don't put the cap on the bottle. Let all the ideas come out.

After you've listed everything that flowed from your mind, you will now be able to look at these ideas in a new light. You will weigh them for their worth in freeing up your time. Remember that the time you have liberated is going to allow you to create a new, richer, fuller, and more satisfying life. That fact alone makes taking the time to do these exercises well worth the effort.

RESOURCE BOX

If you would like to read about some "generic" simplification ideas, you might try one of Elaine St. James' very practical books: *Simplify Your Life, Inner Simplicity* and *Living the Simple Life.*

As you complete each KEEPER #4—MY (AREA OF LIFE) ACTIVITIES, you need to figure out how much time you will save with your ideas for change. Take another look at the examples on pages 169 and 172 which show how to calculate "total cultural time" and "cultural percent time."

Then, calculate the annual hours corresponding to each activity you choose to underline in the right-hand columns of MY (AREA OF LIFE) ACTIVITIES sheets. Now add them up to get the total time for each area. Finally, calculate the new percentage time for each area, based on the simplifications you have decided upon.

Congratulations! Although you probably haven't reached the 20 percent goal for each Area of Life, I'll bet you have made tremendous progress. To help you celebrate and get a fix on just how much progress you've made, fill in your percentages on the following chart and find the total.

YOUR NEW ALLOCATION OF TIME

Area of Life	The Ideal "You"	The Old "You"	Work-In-Progress "You"
Cultural	20%	%	%
Mental	20%	%	%
Physical	20%	%	%
Social	20%	%	%
Spiritual	20%	%	%
TOTALS	100%	100%	%

The grand total for the "Work-In-Progress You" will not add up to 100% because you have reduced or eliminated some activities completely. To see just how much time you have freed up, subtract the "Work-In-Progress You" total from 100%. WOW! When was the last time you had the potential of that much free time on your hands?

Don't go wasting away that time now. We're going to put it to <u>really good use</u> in Part 3. There you'll see how to create a future of success, happiness, and fulfillment for yourself.

For right now, though, you have really accomplished a lot! All of that introspection and self awareness, all of that communicating with your subconscious, and all of those calculations, are finally about to pay off. You are on the brink of taking control of your life. You are about to take the steps that will advance the course of your life forever.

Believe it or not, the rest of the way is all downhill. You have already finished the grunt work: You have cleared away the clutter. You have your road map in hand, and the direction in which you want to take your life is becoming clear. Now you're ready to select the road you want to travel as you begin your journey to a new life.

✛

Part 3

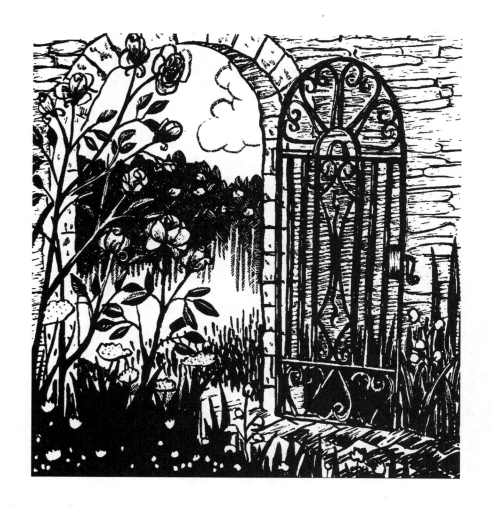

Taking Control of
Your Life

Part 3

INTRODUCTION

Taking Control of Your Life

In Part 3 you will take control of your life and begin realizing the benefits you have been looking for. Your future happiness, good health, wealth and wisdom is just up the road—you can almost see it from here.

You will take contol by interweaving the following processes:

1. making plans for your future and

2. acquiring an accurate perspective on problems that are common in each Area of Life.

The process of making plans involves the step-by-step procedures in three chapters:

- Chapter 7 will review your creations from Chapters 2 and 3 (KEEPERS #1 & 2) to distinguish between your PURPOSE, GOALS and ACTIONS. The result will be a clear definition of your PURPOSE and the categorization of some of your GOALS and ACTIONS into the five Areas of Life.

- Chapter 8 will review your results from Chapters 4-6 (KEEPERS #3-5) to finalize your GOAL for each Area of Life and support it with worthwhile ACTIONS. These will be your Plans for each Area of Life.

- Chapter 9 will use your Plan for each Area of Life to prioritize, schedule and monitor your future ACTIONS in order to achieve your GOALS and realize your PURPOSE.

Each step of the way you will experience additional benefits such as the joy of doing what you want to do, the satisfaction of realizing your dreams, the self-respect of being your own person and the recognition that you are fulfilling your potential.

The process of gaining an <u>accurate perspective</u> on problem areas that trouble many people involves

1   answering a few questions about your own life to determine if you personally have any of the problems which many people share in each Area of Life,

2   reading the discussion dealing with the problems that you need to review, and

3   incorporating your new perspective on these common problems into your GOALS and ACTIONS for each Area of Life.

The sections dealing with Area of Life problems and perspectives are contained <u>within</u> Chapter 8. You will find the following sub-chapters:

- 8A--How to Enjoy a Healthy Physical Life (*Climate: Weathering It's Effects*),

- 8B--How to Enjoy a Wise Spiritual Life (*Spirituality: What It Is and What It Isn't*),

- 8C--How to Enjoy a Healthy Mental Life (*Job Stress: Spotting and Beating This Occupational Hazard*),

- 8D--How to Enjoy a Happy Social Life (*Relationships: Finding and Hanging onto "Good People"*),

- 8E--How to Enjoy a Wealthy Cultural Life (*Careers: Identifying the "Right Job" for You*) and (*Money: Making and Keeping Enough Legally to Be Set Financially*).

In other words, these two processes are intertwined in Chapter 8 so that you can be assured the GOALS and ACTIONS making up your Plan will be certain to reflect the correct perspective on the most common problems that people experience in each of the Areas of Life. Only then will you experience a new sense of inner peace and self confidence as you take control of your life.

"The purpose of life
is
a life of purpose."

—Robert Byrne

Chapter 7

How to Support Your Purpose
with
Meaningful Goals

People who are happy and successful have a clear vision of their PURPOSE. This vision reflects

    1. who they are, and

    2. why they are here.

They support this PURPOSE with GOALS that they have the time, energy and motivation to achieve in each Area of Life. These people then support their GOALS with ACTIONS, ACTIONS they are not afraid to undertake.

Whether you arrived at this point in the book by working your way through Parts 1 and 2, or just by working through KEEPERS #1-5, you're now ready to take control of your life. How? By steering it in the direction you want: your PURPOSE supported by GOALS supported by ACTIONS.

In this chapter you will:

- Take stock of who you are and why you are here. You will then be able to define your PURPOSE for being on Earth. Knowing your PURPOSE will root out any feelings of worthlessness you may be carrying around. It will also fill you with a sense of inner peace and instill you with a joy of living.

• Review your "do something" ideas for overcoming your fears, and your "ideas for change" to simplify and balance your life. This will prepare you to begin setting GOALS and taking ACTION that will give structure to your "ideas" for improving your future. It is this structure that will enable you to conquer any troublesome feelings of helplessness you may have, and replace them with the satisfaction and control you desire.

• Then you will record all this important information on KEEPER #6—MY PURPOSE WORKSHEET.

"It's never too late
to be
who you might
have been."

Look how far you've come. By the time you start reading this chapter, you should already have:

- an understanding of who you are and why you're here.

- thrown away your excuses for not taking action and begun to overcome your fears.

- identified how to simplify the way you live by balancing your life.

However, you HAVE NOT yet started to use the many methods successful people use to take control of their lives. You are ready to take control of your life, but you haven't started yet. That's the aim of this chapter—to coach you through the steps you <u>must</u> take to become the master of your own destiny.

When was the last time you felt like you were in the driver's seat, aiming your life where you wanted it to go? Maybe you never have experienced that sense of controlled direction. If not, get ready for one of the most energizing, one of the most exhilarating feelings in the world. You're about to take the steps necessary to put you behind the wheel. You will be fully equipped with the tools to create and follow your own map toward future happiness and fulfillment.

Before you begin, let me give you the "keys to the car:" a PURPOSE supported by GOALS supported by ACTIONS. It's been the secret of success for years. Organizations and individuals alike use it. You can, too.

TABLE V

How to Take Control of Your Life

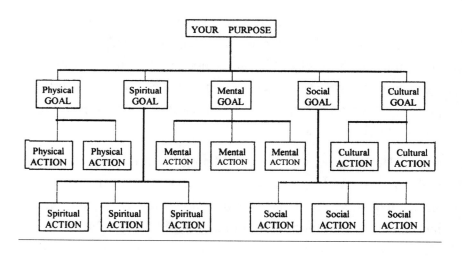

So, How Does the Process Work?

You've already taken the time and effort to understand who you are and why you are here. That's good. But you have to put this knowledge to use. If you don't, you could spend the rest of your life just floundering—never fulfilling your purpose or your potential.

Is that how you want to be remembered? I'll bet not. But it could happen. Think of all the dreamers you know—people who spout with great enthusiasm how they are going to "be this" or "do that." They then drift and meander and never come close to living their grandiose dreams. It's not necessarily because they don't really want to do it. More often, it's because they don't know how to map out the road they want to travel in order to succeed.

My niece, "Chris", is in a bind like that. She has a great deal of natural artistic ability. Her father is a talented artist who has encouraged her interest and creativity since she was a child.

Chris even has an artistic temperament. She spends all of her spare time on creative projects and has never talked or dreamed of becoming anything else. She graduated from a fine California art college. Chris was full of enthusiasm for her purpose of bringing people, places, and things to life with her drawings and paintings so others could enjoy them.

However, years after completing her formal education, she still works at two libraries in order to make ends meet. (That's a job she started so she could make enough money to pay for college.) She has earned next to nothing as an artist. Even worse, she appears no closer to doing so now than the day she graduated several years ago.

Has her dream changed? Does she have another purpose? Not at all! Chris just doesn't know how to go about fulfilling her purpose. She doesn't have the tools needed to put her talents and abilities to work so she can experience her most important mission in life. Like many others, she knows why she is here, but she doesn't know <u>what</u> to do or <u>how</u> to do it.

Let's make sure your major mission in life doesn't get stalled that way. For starters, let's make sure you understand the importance of setting goals which support your purpose. Here it is: You'll never get any closer to your missions in life if you don't establish very specific goals for yourself in each Area of Life. Your goals define <u>what</u> you will do to realize your purpose.

Goals alone won't do the job, however. You have to marry goals to positive actions which will carry them out. That's the only way to bring yourself closer to achieving your goals.

Incidentally, these actions aren't great galloping leaps. They're small steps, one after another. That's the way all significant projects get completed. Your action plans define <u>how</u> you will accomplish your goals.

Successful people (and you're in the process of becoming one) define their purposes and set goals just as successful businesses do. General Motors didn't become one of the most successful companies of the 20th century just because its management had a dream.

The management of American Motors (ever heard of them?) probably had a similar dream. That auto company doesn't exist anymore—nor do its cars, the Nash, Hornet, Gremlin, or Rambler. Why?

It takes more than a dream, more than a purpose, and more than knowing <u>why</u> you are here. It also takes the creation of specific goals—realistic targets that define <u>what</u> you will do to come closer to your purpose.

-To illustrate-

GM's PURPOSE (<u>why</u> it exists): *create wealth for its owners by satisfying the driving needs of people around the world with quality automobiles at competitive prices.*

GM's GOALS (<u>what</u> it will do):

- achieve an above average (12%) annual return on GM common stock,

- become a presence in the auto market of every industrialized country,

- build manufacturing plants where markets dictate and economies of scale are beneficial, providing jobs locally,

- engineer with economically feasible technology which keep the vehicles competitive,

- control the quality of vehicles produced by subjecting them to extensive testing, and

- establish a dealer network with appropriate incentives for superior performance.

If you don't have specific goals to identify what you must do to fulfill your purpose, your dream will fade into oblivion. Are you willing to let your future deteriorate the way the management of American Motors let its company collapse? I didn't think so!

Notice that these goals explain only _what_ will be done, not _how_ it will be done. The "hows" are the ACTIONS that enable you to reach the GOALS.

For example, to achieve its financial goal of 12% average annual return to investors, GM might plan to pay out a stock dividend of 4%. They could accomplish the rest of the goal by growing the price of the stock. Just as you should have several goals to support your mission, you should have several actions to support each goal.

You may be tempted to skip the step of setting goals and try going directly to the actions themselves. Don't. I repeat, DON'T. Your goals are part of your road map. If you have no map, you won't know where you're going and you won't have any idea how to get there. It's likely you will wind up going around in a circle or hitting one dead end after another.

You've probably already done that. That's why you're reading this book and using this process to take control of your life. It's your GOALS which will guarantee you're going in a direction consistent with your purpose in life. First you have to establish goals. Only then can you realistically identify actions that will enable you to aim and move your life in the direction you want to go.

If you have any confusion about this process, take another look at the diagram in Table V. It tells the whole story.

TABLE V

How to Take Control of Your Life

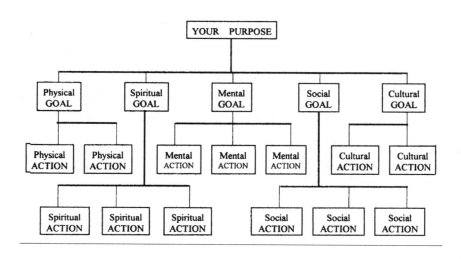

Now, take a deep breath, then exhale.

You're ready to take the next step: reviewing what you have learned about yourself so far. You've done a lot to prepare yourself to take control of your life. Let's make sure the results of your efforts are in the forefront of your mind as you get ready to think about your PURPOSE, GOALS and ACTIONS. If you put them together properly, your troubles will begin to disappear as you use the keys to your car to drive where you want to go.

First, let's look back down the road you've traveled to get here. You took one of two routes.

Some of you read through Part 1: Understanding Yourself and Part 2: Removing Obstacles from Your Life. As you read these chapters, you took each step laid out to prepare you to make changes in your life. In the process, you created five very important personal documents—KEEPERS #1-5. There, you summarized who you are, why you are here, what you can do to overcome your fears and what you can do to simplify and balance your life.

Others of you took a different route and could bypass one or more chapters because your diagnostic Self-Tests results said to skip them. You too, however, have documented your thoughts about yourself and your ideas for the future directly on KEEPERS #1-5. Let's review what those Keepers are about:

#1-MY RESOURCES—The Highlights of My Personality,

#2-MY MISSION STATEMENTS,

#3-MY "DO SOMETHING" IDEAS to Confront My Fears,

#4-MY (AREA OF LIFE) ACTIVITIES—"Ideas for Change,"

#5-MY WHEEL OF BALANCE.

Stop right here if you somehow managed to get to this part of the book without completing all these KEEPERS! Now is the time to go into the KEEPER Forms Section and finish them. Only then will you be ready to make <u>positive</u> changes in your life.

Please don't cheat yourself. Regardless of how well you may know who you are and why you are here, regardless of how fearless you may be, regardless of how simple and well balanced your life may be, you need to concentrate on each of these aspects of your life for a few minutes *before* going any further.

The introspection these KEEPERS guide you through, help pave the road on which you will travel into your future of happiness, good health, wealth and wisdom. You would not want to run the risk of driving a great distance in a car with three bald tires and a temperamental transmission, would you? Well, this is more important than any car you've ever driven. This is <u>your life</u> we're talking about.

When you have finished KEEPERS #1-5, it's time to get on with the next step.

Step 1: Finding the Peace of Mind that Accompanies PURPOSE

This step is a review of KEEPERS #1 & #2—a review you should make while thinking about your PURPOSE, your GOALS and your ACTION plans. For example, as you think about the contents of KEEPER #1—MY RESOURCES, you should ask yourself

● Do my purpose and goals emphasize my strengths and accept my limitations?

● Do my purpose and goals allow me to participate in the activities I enjoy most and the roles I prefer to play?

● Do my purpose and goals embody my strongest beliefs and also the most important principles that guide my life?

If you came up with any "no" answers, you need to do some work on your PURPOSE. You need to make sure that your reason for being here is a true reflection of who you are. KEEPER #1—MY RESOURCES is an accurate picture of YOU. To lead a happy and successful life, your purpose and goals must be compatible with who you are.

For example, my son's goal of becoming a physical therapist was totally consistent with who he is. He has always been at ease with people and very astute at diagnosing problems. Exercise and physical activities have always been important to him He strongly believes in the power of medical science. And, he has been guided by a strong sense of service to others ever since he was small. This is who he is. Becoming a physical therapist allowed him to BE who he is.

On the other hand, my cousin was unhappy when she did what she set out to do: becoming a wife and mother. She was miserable because what she had to do as a wife and mother was not particularly compatible with her personality.

My cousin may be intelligent, but she is not domestically inclined. She prefers to relate to people on an adult basis involving "grown-up" activities. She's very comfortable advising people, but not supervising them. One of her most important guiding principles is independence, both in herself and others.

Obviously, she didn't review her "Personality Highlights" before deciding to try parenthood. Fortunately, she later paid great attention to her personality when she made her "mid-life correction." She pursued both a divorce and a master's degree to have a career in guidance counseling.

When you reflect upon your purpose and your goals, remember that only on very rare occasions does your career turn out to be your PURPOSE. Very few jobs or careers can measure up to the high ideals of a purpose.

For example, just as General Motors' purpose is not merely "making automobiles," your purpose is not merely driving a bus or programming software or being a nurse or managing an office. GM's purpose is "to create wealth for its owners by satisfying the driving needs of people around the world with quality automobiles at competitive prices." What's your PURPOSE?

Your PURPOSE is probably one of your missions that you recorded on KEEPER #2. As such, it involves:

- playing a role or roles for the benefit of others,

- by using your strengths and talents,

- while being guided by your most important principles.

However, your PURPOSE is not just any mission. It is your most important mission. Your purpose is **your life's work**. Everything else in your life either prepares you for your purpose or supports your purpose. I repeat: Your purpose is **your life's work**. Everything else in your life either prepares you for your purpose or supports your purpose.

As you review KEEPER #2—MY MISSION STATEMENTS, ask yourself

- Does this mission qualify as my life's work or is this really preparation for my purpose?

- Does this mission meet the standard of being my purpose in life, or is it more of a supporting goal?

If what you have on KEEPER #2 appears to be more of a goal, record it as such in the appropriate spot on KEEPER #6—MY PURPOSE WORKSHEET.

For example, your career is probably a cultural goal to support your purpose. That shouldn't be surprising. Your physical, mental, social and spiritual goals should also support your purpose.

We saw that General Motors has several goals in support of its purpose; you need to have multiple goals to support your purpose in life. In GM's case, the management must ensure that each of the "functions" of the business are working together to bring the purpose to reality. In your case, you need to make sure that you have a goal for each Area of Life which supports your primary reason for being here.

If you think about GM's goals, you find that the first is a financial one, the second marketing, next manufacturing, then engineering, followed by quality control, and finally distribution. None of these functions of the business can have a goal which is incompatible with GM's overall purpose: to create wealth for its owners by satisfying the driving needs of people around the world with quality automobiles at competitive prices. Having just one part of the business out of synch with the overall purpose could ruin the entire enterprise.

Apparently, that's what happened to American Motors. I'd bet the engineering goal was the culprit there. Have you ever seen an American Motors Gremlin? It looked just as ugly as its name.

But I'm not trying to sell you a car. I'm trying to help you understand the importance of creating a goal for each Area of Life, a goal which supports your purpose. To do that, you must pay attention to your Spiritual life and also your Social, Mental, Physical, and Cultural goals. So, begin recording some of your goals from KEEPER #2 onto KEEPER #6—MY PURPOSE WORKSHEET.

You have to take this step so that the path you create will lead you toward your purpose. If you don't, your life will head off in directions you don't intend and you will end up doing things you don't want to do. It's hard enough to stay on track when your goals in the five areas are all compatible. If you let one or two areas slip, you'll find yourself headed in directions you didn't expect or want.

To help identify your real PURPOSE, it is beneficial to focus on the principles that you consider being vital to your existence. Table VI contains a partial list of guiding virtues that many happy and successful people have adopted.

TABLE VI

Personal Principles

Caring	Contribution
Devotion	Humility
Industry	Integrity
Love	Moderation
Reciprocity	Service
Sharing	Simplicity
Thrift	Trust

Don't be bashful. Go ahead and add some of your own strongest principles to the list. For the next 15 minutes, just free associate and write them down. After you've finished, pick the four that are most important to you. Your PURPOSE will involve one or more of these four guiding virtues in your life.

Now take another pass at KEEPER #2—MY MISSION STATEMENTS. Any mission statements that don't measure up to your highest-order principles are actually goals. They may be very important goals that are essential to your realizing your purpose, but they are not your PURPOSE.

Any of your mission statements that do measure up, however, are candidates for being your PURPOSE. It's even possible that your purpose is something you might have overlooked when you were writing down your mission statements. So keep an open mind about what your PURPOSE is.

Consider this: It is not unusual if your spiritual mission turns out to be your high PURPOSE. In fact, that's exactly what happened to me. Midway through my career in the organizational world, I was convinced my purpose was to be an organizational planner. I based that decision on my analytical abilities and experience in industry, government, and education.

I was guided by the principle of being of help to as many people as possible. As I look back, though, my spiritual goals—finding and sharing the wisdom of life—never supported this purpose. Organizations are rarely interested in the wisdom of life. They are interested in their own purpose, the perpetuation of their own existence and succeeding in much more material terms, such as amassing money or power.

I was at cross-purposes with the organizations. Consequently, my perfectly admirable purpose of organizational planning was doomed to fail—and did! Fortunately, I was able to recover in time. I pursued my real reason for being here after I discovered what it was. Here it is:

USING MY ANALYTICAL SKILLS AND OBJECTIVE PERSPECTIVE ON LIFE, I WILL BE A COUNSELOR AND COACH TO MY CLIENTS, STUDENTS, FAMILY AND FRIENDS. I WILL DO THIS WHILE BEING GUIDED BY A STRONG SENSE OF DEVOTION AND INTEGRITY.

As you can see, this purpose is much more spiritual because it involves the principle of devotion and the role of counselor—both spiritual in nature. Perhaps you can learn from my error of mistaking a cultural mission as my PURPOSE. Look toward your spiritual mission when you are searching for your purpose in life. Whether or not you find your PURPOSE there, your spiritual mission certainly is a productive place to look.

At this point you need to write down on KEEPER #6—MY PURPOSE WORKSHEET exactly what you believe your purpose to be. Remember not to confuse this most important mission with other missions that are really just a means to your end. For example, in my case, my career in the organizational world was not my purpose. It turned out to be only financial and educational preparation for my real purpose in life.

But you've got to make the effort. It's necessary for you to do what every other happy and successful person has already done. If you are to join them, you must explore not only who you are but also why you're here. Once you unearth your reason for being here, you can leave behind the life that didn't work. It will be like taking off clothing that didn't fit. It cloaked you with discomfort and left you feeling disheartened and confused.

Now you must pick out new clothing for yourself, suited to your taste and temperament. When you put it on, it will fit you just right. So you have to commit yourself to picking the outfit—the purpose—that fits you, that makes you feel and be your best.

RESOURCE BOX

If you are having trouble deciding what your purpose is, take a step back and ask yourself
1) What is worthy of my time, energy and talents?
2) What are my hopes and dreams for the future?

KEEPER #6

MY PURPOSE WORKSHEET

My Purpose in Life is to use my _____ to
(traits and talents)

be a _____ guided by _____,
(role)   (principles)

for the benefit of _____.
(recipients)

	Goals	Actions
Physical		
Mental		
Social		
Spiritual		
Cultural		

Step 2: Creating Self-Satisfaction by Adding Structure to Your Life

Ultimately, you need to define a goal in each Area of Life that will support your PURPOSE. A GOAL is a target that you think you can realistically reach. You may not know how to get there just yet, but that's not important right now. The important thing is that <u>attaining your goal will facilitate your **being** who your PURPOSE says you are.</u>

For example, remember my purpose: *USING MY ANALYTICAL SKILLS AND OBJECTIVE PERSPECTIVE ON LIFE, I WILL BE A COUNSELOR AND COACH TO MY CLIENTS, STUDENTS, FAMILY AND FRIENDS. I WILL BE GUIDED BY A STRONG SENSE OF DEVOTION AND INTEGRITY.*

In support of my purpose, I had the following cultural, mental, physical, social and spiritual goals:

- CULTURAL: Attain a position of financial independence so I can "retire" from the organizational world at an age young enough to pursue my primary mission in life.

- MENTAL: Get to know myself objectively in terms of my traits, beliefs and principles, and also the impact on me by other people's behavior and the changes occurring in society.

- PHYSICAL: Maintain my good health and physical conditioning, free from any addictive substances.

- SOCIAL: Provide a secure and stable home for my family so our children will feel free to "return" while getting oriented into the cultural worlds of higher education and work.

- SPIRITUAL: Become a "wise" person who has life in perspective and can advise others on how to make progress toward their desired personal objectives.

Notice that these statements <u>are not</u> mission statements. They don't identify any traits or talents that I will be using. They don't specify any roles that I will be playing. They don't enumerate any principles that will guide me. However, these statements <u>are</u> goals. *They are targets I believe are reachable, which makes it easier for me to realize my purpose.* They don't explain <u>how</u> I will accomplish the results (ACTIONS), they only define <u>what</u> I am shooting for (GOALS).

"When you act as you
wish yourself to be,
in due course,
you become as you act."

—Norman Vincent Peale

See how Table V is beginning to evolve as I took control of my life.

TABLE V

How to Take Control of Your Life

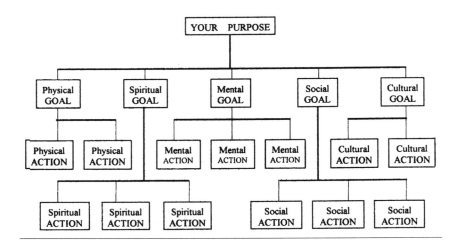

I have defined my PURPOSE. I have also set five GOALS, one for each Area of Life to facilitate my PURPOSE. The next step is to specify ACTION plans that will enable me to accomplish my GOALS.

As you revisit KEEPER #3—MY "DO SOMETHING" IDEAS to Confront My Fears, and KEEPER #4—MY (AREA OF LIFE) ACTIVITIES—"Ideas for Change," pay particular attention to which of your "ideas" are GOALS and which are ACTIONS. Remember, GOALS are where you want to go. ACTIONS are what you will do to get there.

Then, write down these ideas for improving your life into the appropriate category of KEEPER #6—MY PURPOSE WORKSHEET. It is the classification of these ideas that will help you to reap the benefits of taking control of your own life.

For example, if one of your "do something" ideas is to lose five pounds per month, that is a physical GOAL. If one of your "do something" ideas is to jog every day, that is a physical ACTION which will help you achieve your goal of losing five pounds each month. Goals specify <u>what</u> you will do. Actions define <u>how</u> you will do it.

My workshop participant, Betty, decided she wanted to simplify her cultural activities. She identified a cultural GOAL (<u>what</u> she will change) when she decided to cut back on the amount of network television she was watching. Her plan to watch only four programs she liked the most each week represents a cultural ACTION (<u>how</u> she will change).

By categorizing your good ideas from Part 2 into goals and actions for each Area of Life, you will be incorporating them into your plans for the future. This is the next step to confronting your fears and carrying out your simplification ideas. Here is a real opportunity for you to use your "DO SOMETHING" IDEAS to face the gremlins that have been standing in the way of your success and happiness.

When I wrote down my cultural financial goal almost 25 years ago, I was as frightened as you probably are now about ongoing financial responsibilities. How was I going to pay the bills for food, a house, my children's college education? But I stood up to that fear by establishing a target I was prepared to shoot for. You must, repeat, <u>must</u> do the same. Challenge your fears!

My niece, "Chris," the aspiring artist, is afraid her work is not good enough to be successful commercially. In addition to tackling that fear by programming her subconscious with a substitute message, she also needs to establish a goal which confronts that fear. For example, she might choose the following cultural goal:

"Conduct an annual exhibit of my art work for public display."

Sure it sounds scary. Remember, though, that during the same time she is striving for this goal, she will continue reprogramming her subconscious to overcome her fear that her work is not good enough.

Of course, she must also create complementary GOALS in her other Areas of Life, then back them up with ACTIONS, all in support of her PURPOSE. If she does, then one day she will **be** what her PURPOSE says she is.

It's that easy! Remember the keys to the car: PURPOSE supported by GOALS supported by ACTIONS. It's the secret of success used by organizations and individuals alike for years.

At this point you have begun to give your life direction. You have defined your PURPOSE on KEEPER #6—MY PURPOSE WORKSHEET. Now you know for sure what you're doing here. You have identified your life's work! You will always have a good reason to get up early in the morning or stay up late at night. Just continue to follow this passion which represents your purpose.

You have also begun to add some structure to your future by classifying your self-improvement ideas into GOALS and ACTIONS in each Area of Life. You will no longer carry around feelings of being helpless. You have identified ways to make your PURPOSE a reality—by deciding <u>what</u> to do and <u>how</u> to do it.

Chapter 8

How to Support Your Goals
with
Worthwhile Actions

Happy and successful people have a realistic outlook on each Area of Life which enables them to avoid or overcome the problems which plague many others. Based on such sound outlooks, these people set realistic GOALS for which they have the motivation to achieve. And they plan relevant ACTIONS that they are not afraid to take to support their PURPOSE in life.

What is your outlook on each Area of Life? In this chapter, you will

- review some specific traps which commonly stop many people—relegating them to an unfulfilled life of frustration, dissatisfaction or even despair. These are traps you may not have thought about. There is at least one major pitfall in each Area of Life. To troubleshoot each of these problems, you'll answer five short questions to determine if you're trapped by any of them.

- read about the happy, healthy, wealthy and wise approach to avoid or escape these traps. There is a helpful perspective on every one of these problems that will show you how to deal with each specific issue.

- sharpen your thinking about your specific problems so you can develop better GOALS and ACTIONS for your Area of Life Plans.

- use KEEPER #7—MY (AREA OF LIFE) PLAN to record your good ideas from KEEPER #6—MY PURPOSE WORKSHEET and the resolution of your perspective in each Area of Life.

- prepare a Self-Talk Tape which explains the importance of your PURPOSE, your GOALS and your ACTIONS to ensure that both your conscious and subconscious mind work together to bring success and fulfillment to your life.

When you complete these steps, you will have KEEPER #7—MY (AREA OF LIFE) PLAN and a Self-Talk Tape that contains the details of your future. Then, you will have the power to control your future. These documents, which you will create in this chapter, are the keys to your self-esteem. They will summarize exactly what you should do and how you should do it to **be** who you really are.

In the previous chapter you began to create some structure in your life by categorizing your GOALS and ACTION plans into each of the five Areas of Life. Before completing this list of GOALS and ACTIONS you need to make certain you are not suffering from any of the problems that stifle many people.

These problems (and there will be at least one from each Area of Life) will be addressed one by one. After a short explanation, you will be asked five questions to detect whether your life is being cramped by that specific problem.

If it is, you should read the discussion on that particular difficulty. Only after reading this perspective should you attempt to complete KEEPER #7—MY (AREA OF LIFE) PLAN for that Area of Life. Only after reading this perspective can you feel certain that

- you possess a healthy outlook and

- any additional GOALS or ACTIONS for that Area of Life will be realistic and appropriate to the support of your PURPOSE.

I know you're probably tempted to start working on the cultural Area of Life first. That's the easiest and the first one that popped into your mind, right? But, remember your KEEPER #5—MY WHEEL OF BALANCE? It's not likely that your cultural area is underweighted. Aren't you already spending too much time there? The last thing you need is a new list of cultural ACTIONS to consume you. Let's move forward.

We're trying to bring your life into balance, not aggravate the imbalances that already exist. So, hold off on the cultural goals and start instead with an Area of Life in which you currently spend less than 20% of your time. If you're going to create a balanced life, one which will give you a smooth ride on your life's journey, now is the time to pump up some of those areas you've neglected.

So, pull out KEEPER #5—MY WHEEL OF BALANCE and consider the Areas of Life in which you need to spend more time. I'm guessing Physical, Mental and Spiritual. It's your choice, but it will help greatly as you proceed if you first review the areas in which you need to be more active. To illustrate the process, I'm going to start with the Physical Area of Life.

Please remember, though, what the objective is here: You need a clear and accurate perspective on each Area of Life so you can understand how to fix any problems in that area. Once you are convinced you have a healthy and realistic outlook, you will use KEEPER #7 to create a plan. This plan will reflect your understanding of any problems in that area.

> "Failing to plan
> is
> planning to fail"
>
> —Benjamin Franklin

SECTION 8A

How to Enjoy a Healthy Physical Life

Many people tend to overlook or at least minimize the impact weather has on us—probably because the weather is something we can't really do anything about. It just happens. If the weather is undesirable—it's raining or sleeting or too hot or too cold—we can always try to stay indoors where the climate is controlled.

However, just because people have modern technological conveniences to make their indoor lives a comfortable shelter from the weather doesn't mean they should become indifferent to it. That's why people spend a significant amount of time talking about the weather, complaining about the weather and trying to "stay on top of the weather." Do you have a realistic understanding of the effects climate has on you, your disposition and your productivity?

Here are five questions relating to this major element of your physical environment. After you answer them, you can decide for yourself if you need to read the following perspective on climate before completing MY PHYSICAL PLAN. (Answer "yes," "no" or "maybe" based on your current geographical location.)

1   Do I usually enjoy the weather where I live?

2   Does the weather make me feel energized?

3   Does the climate contribute to my well-being?

4   Does the climate have a positive effect on me?

5   Am I healthier living here rather than in some other climate?

If you honestly answered YES to four or five of these questions, please skip the following explanation of climate and its effect on human behavior. You aren't troubled by the common misconception that the weather doesn't bother you. You're ready to create KEEPER #7—MY PHYSICAL PLAN.

But, if two or more of your responses were NO, or "maybe" or even "sometimes," then I urge you to read the following perspective before tackling MY PHYSICAL PLAN.

Climate: Weathering its Effects

Pity your ancestors. They were at the mercy of the climate. They were sweaty and sunburned in summer, whipped by winter gales and blizzards in the winter. You're much better off. You probably have central heating and air conditioning in your home and your workplace. You have a climate control system in your car. Modern technology has smoothed out many of the temperature and humidity extremes your ancestors had to tolerate.

This does not mean climate no longer affects you. To the contrary, climate changes are one of the biggest forces shaping how you think, act and feel. Many factors are so subtle that you're likely to downplay or even ignore the profound effects they have on your life. Don't worry, you have plenty of company. Even doctors and psychologists who attempt to explain individual differences often overlook how climate shapes us.

Some people don't have to think about it. They know very well; they know down deep in their bones. Ask people suffering from arthritis about the effects of barometric pressure changes on their joints. Or ask an asthmatic about the wind and what happens when it changes speed and direction. Talk to someone who has a skin condition about the effects of humidity or the lack of it.

The life-cramping effects of these reactions to the climate are why people talk about being "under the weather" and staying "on top of the weather."

This perspective will give you some information so you can do a better job of staying " on top of the weather" by

- understanding how climate effects you,

- setting your Physical GOAL accordingly, and

- including a Physical action plan to move to a more favorable area, if that's appropriate.

Actually, people react to their climates in ways that go far beyond just physical symptoms. Climate can hit people hard, altering even their moods, emotions, dreams and perceptions. Climate can alter the way you think and can even distort or magnify parts of your personality.

Climate and weather patterns also help mold how you interact with other people. If you do a lot of business on the phone, you've probably noticed how seldom your phone rings when a storm is approaching. The sky is overcast, and a pressure system is developing. When gloomy weather begins to appear, people want to deal with the change in weather. They isolate themselves and busy themselves with projects they have "saved for a rainy day" instead of making sales calls or engaging in tricky negotiations.

Warm, sunny, dry days, are just the opposite. That's when most people are much more likely to phone business contacts or visit them in person. The energy bursts people seem to get from good weather help to launch new projects. When people are feeling good, they're more likely to contact others instead of keeping to themselves.

These same principles apply equally to large group interactions. For example, research has correlated extended droughts with the start of wars. It's not because these prolonged dry spells bring hardship and scarcity. It's because hardship and scarcity produce instability and fear. Often, societies, seeing that a drought threatens their way of life, are willing to sustain themselves by waging war on other people. In this same way, major swings in the world economic markets have been correlated with major climatic changes.

Once you understand the influence of the climate on your health and your behavior, you can probably reduce your medical bills. For example, feelings of depression, being sluggish and "down," aren't necessarily some kind of permanent abnormality. In fact, such feelings can be a normal product of the natural impact of weather conditions on you. Every cell in your body must adapt to weather changes. If those changes are too extreme or too frequent for you to keep up with them, you experience stress—climatic stress.

That brings us to the main point of understanding how the climate surrounding you—from the air you breathe to the number of rainy and snowy days you endure—affects you. If you want to reduce the stress of these factors, I have some news. The only permanent solution is to make a big change. You must find a new climate in which to live. You need to move.

Of course, that isn't always possible. There are tradeoffs. But, in the long run, anything is possible. Meanwhile, at least you should try to maximize the energizing effects of the weather where you do live and to minimize the damaging consequences.

SOME MEDICAL EVIDENCE

The effect of climate and weather on humans has been recognized by medical science for a long time. Around 400 BC, Hippocrates said that "melancholia occurs in the spring." And, everyone is familiar with the term "spring fever."

Moving can have its own medical consequences. If you move to a new area with weather patterns different from the ones you're used to, you'll have to go through a process of acclimation. Your biochemistry must adapt to the influences of your new surroundings before you begin to feel "normal" again. Inevitably, you'll go through a short period of adjustment when you won't feel quite yourself. You'll feel vaguely uneasy and somewhat "out of sync."

Some individuals adjust to climate changes very easily. Others are far more sensitive. If you live in a place where the four seasons are very pronounced, you already know how quickly you adjust to the changing seasons. Some people have trouble adapting to the dark, dreary winter days and flourish mightily in the bright, sunny summer. Medical science now says that people whose temperament becomes melancholy during the winter suffer from seasonal affective disorder (SAD).

The symptoms of SAD include:

- depression,

- irritability and anxiety,

- increases in appetite and weight,

- longer periods of sleep,

- drowsiness during the day,

- decreased sex drive,

- difficulty at work, and

- troublesome interpersonal relations.

Although you probably don't suffer from SAD, you may have noticed that you're more likely to have one or more of these symptoms during months when the sunshine is rare or the weather changes dramatically from day to day.

You shouldn't be surprised. Nature has plenty of tipoffs that this situation exists. Many plant varieties are totally dormant during the winter months and then blossom during the spring and summer. The bear is just one example of the many animal species which hibernate during the winter. The rest of the year, the bear forages, mates, tends its young and plays in the sunshine.

Our lives are not so measured. We don't have the luxury of a life cycle giving us time off to sleep for several months. We're expected to function year-round. Maybe during some point in our evolution we did get to take a long winter's nap. No more. We are expected to be at top speed and top efficiency no matter what time of year it is or what the weather is doing outside.

We do have some things in common with the bear and other animals. Scientists have detected a hormone which animals' brains produce during winter months. It's called melatonin. Research has shown that shorter days and decreased sunlight cause the human brain to produce melatonin, too.

These findings help explain why individuals who succumb to SAD have reported that their problems are noticeably relieved when they travel closer to the equator. Scientists now are experimenting with increased year-round heat and light for moderating the symptoms of SAD. Because heat can already be controlled quite well by most Westerners—central climate control and a thermostat are pretty handy inventions—most of the studies have concentrated on increasing the patient's exposure to light.

To date, experiment results show that extending the periods of normal indoor lighting won't do the trick. Having high-intensity lighting (ten times normal) for six hours per day, however, does suppress melatonin production, thus reversing a patient's depression and associated symptoms.

Take heed. The results of this research and the related ways in which animals adapt to seasonal changes should motivate you to take a closer look at your climate when considering the physical influences in your life.

RESOURCE BOX

Climate also affects the way groups behave. Changes in weather patterns particularly affect the actions of political parties and financial institutions. Climatologist Dr. Iben Browning looks at time in terms of millions of years. He has shown that when the cycles of the sun and tide converge, volcanoes start to rumble. The amount of dust from volcanic eruptions can be enough to blot out the sun's rays, cooling the earth. Browning concluded that recessions, depressions, and the fall of governments happen when the sun's effects are blocked by volcanic dust. The more volcanoes spitting ashes into the air, the more likely it is that economies and governments will fall.

A STRATEGY FOR PRODUCTIVITY & FULFILLMENT

What does all this mean to you? Well, in order to lead a fulfilling existence, you must recognize the importance of climate and weather patterns in your life. They can be as significant a part of your environment as your friends, your family, the media, your teachers and your employer. Weather patterns influence your thoughts, your moods and your physical well-being.

You should reflect upon which climate conditions are best and worst for you. Only after you understand the climate's personal effect can you plan a strategy taking this important environmental influence into account.

One way to help you get a handle on this issue is to ask yourself: During which months of the year am I the happiest? If you begin to see a seasonal pattern emerging, you are probably safe in drawing the correlation between feeling good and weather patterns.

Most people are happiest during the months of June, July, and December. The reasons have to do with both the climate and social conditions. June and July are favorable because the weather is good in most areas and because many people take their vacations at that time. December, of course, has such an uplifting holiday season that for many people even the dreariest winter weather seems filled with sunshine.

If you can pinpoint the climate that brings out the best in you, you should set your GOALS accordingly. On a long-term basis, this means planning to live in a climate that energizes you. If rain gives you a burst of energy, plan to relocate or, at least retire, to an area which gets more than its fair share. The Pacific Northwest would be terrific for you. On the other hand, sun worshipers who suffer depression during the passage of major low pressure systems (rain, storms or unsettled air) will want to head for the temperate deserts of the southwestern U.S.

On a short-term basis, though, such relocations aren't usually possible. The best you can do is schedule your activities to coincide with the weather conditions. Of course you already know not to schedule a picnic when it rains. Similarly, you should try to schedule the final stages of an important financial transaction when the climate is the most energizing for you. This action will probably increase your chances of doing well in that deal. Scheduling your life, when possible, to coincide with the climate's beneficial effects on you, will make you more productive and more fulfilled.

One final point regarding the weather: Don't get frustrated and grouchy when you're not feeling your best! The reason just might be the weather, and you have absolutely no control over that. The only way to deal with the weather is what you've learned during this review:

1   Understand how climate effects you.

2   Set your Physical GOAL accordingly.

3   Plan to relocate to a more favorable area if appropriate.

You should now have in focus the perspective that climate is one of the most significant parts of your physical environment, both directly and indirectly. On a direct basis, it can either charge you up or drain your batteries, depending on your physical makeup. You are also subject to weather conditions indirectly because you, like everybody else, are subject to unfolding economic and political events around the world. These events are, to some extent, determined by weather patterns. Remember:

1. You can't control the weather, but you can minimize the stress that it causes you. You can try to schedule your activities so that what you do coincides with how you're feeling:

- Be engaged in important, productive tasks when the climate energizes you.

- Fiddle with busy work when the weather drains you.

2. You can make a commitment in your long-range planning to relocate or retire to a more favorable climate when the opportunity presents itself. You may not be able to control the weather, but you should view it as an important influence on your physical health.

3. When you create MY PHYSICAL PLAN, climate should be included as something that enhances your life, not something you have to tolerate and try to "stay on top of."

4. The weather does not need to be a problem as long as you accept that it can greatly affect your comfort and physical health.

Step 1: How to Create MY PHYSICAL PLAN

Now that you have some new information about the climate, it's time to create your overall plan for the Physical Area of Life.

The process of establishing a plan for any Area of Life involves focusing totally on that aspect of your existence. What are the things that bring you a sense of physical well being? Exercise? A good meal? Sunshine? What are the things in life that interfere with your feelings of well being? The flu? The rain? A hangover? In other words, think about the desirable things which make and keep you healthy and the undesirables that lead to poor health.

This assessment has a very practical use. By thinking about these issues you can avoid defining GOALS which will turn out badly for you. You want to create GOALS which will help you to be who you want to be and energize you in the process.

To help with this step, take another look at KEEPER #6—MY PURPOSE WORKSHEET. Review the GOALS and ACTIONS you have already listed for the Physical Area of Life. (Don't forget how important the climate can be to many people, including yourself.)

Now that you are really focused on your physical self, begin filling out KEEPER #7A—MY PHYSICAL PLAN. Jot down the ideas that have been rolling around in your head. Come up with a reachable physical target that five, ten, or 20 years from now will help facilitate your being who you really are. Just use the top of the sheet for your Physical goal as I did on my sample KEEPER #7A. Mine came directly from MY PURPOSE WORKSHEET:

"MAINTAIN MY GOOD HEALTH AND PHYSICAL CONDITIONING, FREE FROM ANY ADDICTIVE SUBSTANCES."

Now let's review how I created an action plan for this GOAL. The most effective way to come up with some ACTIONS that will help you achieve your GOAL is to "meditate on the goal." This is nothing new. You already know how to do that. We've done some meditation from time to time when you had to tap into your subconscious and let it help you. Look back at Chapter 3: Step 3 to remind yourself how, if you need to.

The same process will work here to help you identify ACTIONS that will support your GOALS. Make no mistake, <u>you need to carry out ACTIONS</u> in order to accomplish your GOALS. Only then can you realize your PURPOSE. Only then can you live the life of success, happiness, and fulfillment that you deserve.

A GOAL without ACTIONS which support it is like a leader without followers: It just disappears! Think about it. What good is knowing <u>what</u> you want to do if you don't know <u>how</u> to go about it?

When you have a GOAL and do nothing to make it a reality, you've cheated yourself. What good is opening a bank account if you don't put any money into it? The bank account is worthless! Without ACTIONS, your GOAL is worthless.

Let's figure out how to accomplish that Physical goal you're so excited about. You can think of this meditation as a kind of internal brainstorming. Organizations come up with action plans for their GOALS by getting the responsible parties together and brainstorming ideas in some tranquil setting away from the pressures of everyday business. Your meditation will serve the same end. It gets your subconscious "talking to" your conscious mind as you brainstorm some alternative actions all by yourself.

So do it. Find yourself a quiet place where you won't be interrupted for a while and just meditate on your PURPOSE and your Physical GOAL. Gradually, you will be able to write down several possible ACTIONS to help you accomplish that GOAL. And while you're at it, pin down the best time or conditions for putting your action plans into motion. These are essential and need to be recorded in the "Comments" column next to the corresponding ACTION.

For example, my internal brainstorming several years ago, when our children were in elementary school, resulted in MY PHYSICAL PLAN on page 244. Notice that I've indicated a time or development when it would be particularly attractive to try each ACTION. Pinning down <u>when</u> you are most likely to succeed will help you become more of an opportunist.

After constructing my PHYSICAL PLAN, I was ready to act when one of our children expressed an interest in cross-country skiing. My son's interest was the condition I had waited for to put into motion my possible cross-country skiing ACTION. That action, among others, was designed to support my Physical GOAL. Achieving that GOAL helped me to experience my PURPOSE in life.

RESOURCE BOX

If you have been working with a trusted friend on previous steps, here is another place where two heads can be better than one. He or she can help you brainstorm some ACTIONS that will enable you to reach your GOALS.

Now watch how it's all beginning to fit together.

- First, on KEEPER #6, you defined your PURPOSE and a GOAL for each Area of Life that will enable you to experience that PURPOSE.

- Now, on KEEPER #7A, you are writing down some Physical ACTIONS you can take to make your Physical GOAL a reality.

- Finally, you are recording the best circumstances for taking those Physical ACTIONS in the "Comments" column of KEEPER #7A.

Let's say it together—PURPOSE supported by GOALS supported by ACTIONS.

"The secret of success
is
constancy of purpose."

—Benjamin Disraeli

MY PHYSICAL PLAN

<u>GOAL</u> — (The target for my physical life which will enable me to fulfill my PURPOSE):

To maintain my good health and physical conditioning, free from any addictive substances.

ACTIONS to consider	Comments
1. Take long bicycle rides	When son is ready
2. Try cross-country skiing	If one of kids interested
3. Exercise regularly	Jog evenings or on weekends
4. Join a health club	Possible noontime activity
5. Have neck pain diagnosed	Get physical therapist referral
6. Do more outside with kids	Weekends and vacations
7. Go on walks with wife	Evenings and days off
8. Install central A/C in home	When money has been saved
9.	
10.	
11.	
12.	
13.	

MY PHYSICAL PLAN

<u>GOAL</u> — (The target for my physical life which will enable me to fulfill my PURPOSE):

_____

_____

_____

ACTIONS to consider	Comments
1.	
2.	
3.	
4.	
5.	
6.	
7.	
8.	
9.	
10.	
11.	
12.	
13.	

Now that you've completed the process for the Physical Area of life, you have begun feeling some of the exhilaration that comes from the knowledge that you have begun taking control of your life. Whatever your PURPOSE in life and whatever your Physical GOAL, you have just identified some specific, concrete ACTIONS. These will make your GOAL and your PURPOSE come true. You have taken a giant step toward being in control of your own future.

You are now ready to focus on the next Area of Life, your spiritual being.

"If you don't stand
for something,
you'll fall
for anything."
—Unknown

SECTION 8B

How to Enjoy a Wise Spiritual Life

Spirituality is not what many people think it is. Simply put, it is having faith in forces and ideas which reach beyond pure logic and explanation. The form it takes is highly personal. For you and everyone else, it is represented by your individual system of Principles and Beliefs.

Many people today feel guilty or at least very uneasy about religious matters, including:

- not having a place of worship,

- not being a good churchgoer, or

- not really believing in everything their religion teaches.

Many people don't even like to think about their spirituality. They are afraid they may not be doing what is "right" or what is good for themselves in the long run. For example, what happens after death? Do you have a realistic perspective on your spirituality? Does your belief system form a foundation that you can turn to in times of need?

Here are five questions to help you decide if you should brush up on your spiritual perspective or if you are ready to construct KEEPER #7B—MY SPIRITUAL PLAN.

1   Do I freely exercise my instincts to establish beliefs beyond what I can see, hear, feel, smell and taste?

2   Are my beliefs a source of grounding for me by providing a basis for my thoughts and actions?

3   Am I confident in my belief system?

4   Do I respect myself because of what I believe?

5   Do my beliefs give me peace of mind and a sense of inner tranquility?

If you responded affirmatively to at least four of these questions, you are ready to move directly to the creation of MY SPIRITUAL PLAN. However, two or more "no's" or "maybe's" or "sometimes" and you need to spend a few minutes contemplating the following perspective on spirituality. You will then be able to view this Area of Life as the important, practical and comforting friend that it should be.

Spirituality: Remembering What It Is and What It Isn't

Spirituality is not what you can see or hear or feel but what you instinctively believe. It may have little or no factual basis. Spirituality is not necessarily about believing in God. Of course, most people do believe in a Supreme Being, but that is not a requirement for being spiritual.

Being spiritual means developing and expressing a system of beliefs and a set of principles that extend beyond your own self. You can be spiritual with, or without, an organized religion. Because no one else sees the universe and its mysteries in quite the same way you do, your beliefs form a system of opinions which is unique to you. In other words, your spirituality is very personal just like your physical, mental and social characteristics are yours and yours alone. If the principles of an organized religion sufficiently match your system of beliefs, that religion should provide you with an excellent expression of your spirituality.

In its simplest form, spirituality simply is having faith in forces reaching beyond pure logic and explanation.

YOU FEEL GROUNDED WHEN YOUR SPIRITUALITY IS HEALTHY

Spirituality has extremely practical uses. It lets you deal with any and all unexplained phenomena that you experience. Science is continually widening what we know about our world and the universe. Even so, there will always be holes, both big and small, in that knowledge. Science can't explain <u>all</u> that we experience or contemplate.

You can see that fact in your own life and in the lives of others. Most of us know someone who has had cancer. Scientists have been trying to pry open the secrets of that ugly disease for years. Yet nobody knows the real cause of cancer or why only certain people get it. Despite many theories, there are few indisputable facts. Even so, you, like most others, have probably formed an opinion which represents your belief on the subject. This belief is part of your faith, your leap beyond science and hard facts — part of your spirituality.

Your spirituality also lets you deal with the rest of the world daily. The way you deal with other people on a daily basis reflects the principles most important to you as you attempt to fit into your environment. Some highly regarded principles include such concepts as security, freedom, moderation, integrity and service. Look over your own KEEPER #1—MY RESOURCES to remind yourself of the most important principles that guide your life. They are part of your spirituality.

One very important set of beliefs to which you have already given considerable thought is your place in the world. In other words, your Mission Statements and your PURPOSE are vital parts of your belief system. They represent your vision about how you interact with others.

Perhaps you see yourself as:

- a God-fearing citizen of the USA trying to do the best you can for your family, or

- a nurturing mother or grandmother protecting the helpless infants and curious toddlers, or

- a stress-relieving entertainer who can make everyone laugh and forget their troubles, or

- a truth-seeking scientist trying to find a cure for a life-threatening disease, or

- an average person doing the best you can to bring a little light into the lives of others.

The actual, specific description of "your place in the Universe" is really very personal. It's important to you because it represents a belief that works for you. That belief identifies your reason for being—your essence—and is the basis for your self-esteem. Yes your PURPOSE is an integral part of your spirituality.

Now is an excellent time to reflect on KEEPER #1—MY RESOURCES. That document will help you remember what other beliefs and principles are important to you. They are all part of your spirituality—ideas that are significant to you though you can't see, hear, feel, smell or taste them.

A BELIEF SYSTEM IS COMFORTING

Earthquakes, floods, droughts and epidemics are woven into the entire history of humanity. The lives of thousands, even millions of people have been ruined or destroyed. These disasters also remind people that they do not have control over many life-threatening events.

At such times in history, organized religions have flourished. Why? Because they are very comforting. People whose lives have been ruined feel better believing that the wreckage was brought about by a force which can and does have control over all these tragedies, and whose random destruction defies any rational explanation.

Believing in a power which is beyond rational understanding means that the power, if properly approached, may stop or diminish future disasters, both cosmic and personal.

We associate a Supreme Being and organized religion with spirituality. Your personal belief regarding a Supreme Being is just one of many opinions in your belief system. Since it is not based on factual evidence, it is another facet of your spirituality.

At times when science makes significant inroads toward the unexplained, organized religion tends to be less important in industrial societies. However, there are still many "less developed" cultures in the world that believe in various gods who control the rainfall and sunshine which produce their food supply. Such people have no control over the climate and cannot survive without favorable growing conditions. So, they believe as part of their religion that "someone" does have control, and they try to stay on "his" or "her" good side.

Organized religions also play an important role with respect to the social as well as the physical environment. In particular, most religions prize the need for people to interact peaceably and productively. So religions develop a moral code which followers are expected to practice.

Such codes of ethics take the form of a system of principles which get unanimously adopted. In most Western religions, the prime example is the 10 Commandments. But whatever principles you live by, they are an essential part of your spirituality. You should be conscious of the rules and the virtues that guide you.

Understanding your system of principles is the first step in becoming comfortable with your spirituality. To illustrate, try the following exercise. Which do you value more in the following pairs?

Money	OR	Family
Wisdom	OR	Happiness
Personal Growth	OR	Helping Others
Freedom	OR	Authority
Pleasure	OR	Safety

The selections that you made to some of life's intangibles further define your spirituality. As you can see, your individual system of principles and beliefs goes well beyond the areas outlined in the Ten Commandments.

So, how does a religion and its house of worship fit into this thing called spirituality? Physically, the church, ashram, synagogue, temple or sweat lodge is the place where you go to contemplate your spirituality. It is in this place that you receive suggestions on how to develop the intuitive dimension of your life.

But, it's also a symbol—a symbol of the system of beliefs and principles adopted by its followers. Furthermore, a religion is an organization, a structure of productive individuals managing the "business of religion." That business includes policies, plans, finances, property, rituals, announcements and social functions.

Religions are in the business of helping you to discover your intuitive self. They do this with a prepackaged system of beliefs and principles that you are expected to accept. If you do, praying will provide you with intuitive self expression and inner self development within the bounds of this system. On the other hand, you may prefer to practice your system of beliefs and principles on your own and set your own pace of spiritual growth. Of course, you can try one or the other at different times in your life.

Fortunately, you live in a society which has guaranteed freedom of religion by its constitution. So, it is truly your choice whether you express your spirituality as an individual or within the framework of an existing institution. In fact, some people have even started their own religion!

The Constitution of the United States goes a step further and requires the separation of church and state. This means that the government cannot infringe on the business of religion and the church cannot infringe on the business of the government. This provision ensures a certain balance of power between these two institutions both of which can exert tremendous influence over the lives of so many people.

The net effect is that <u>you</u> are in control of your own spirituality—not the government and not the church. You decide what you believe and you decide what principles guide you. If your beliefs and principles are compatible with an existing religious organization, then you are free to choose to join in the structure and activities of that church.

But, it is your responsibility to find comfort and contentment with your spirituality. If that comfort comes from an established church, you are fortunate. Join it and support it. If, on the other hand, you are more comfortable contemplating your spirituality on your own or among family and friends, you are likewise fortunate. You can handle these matters yourself.

The most important things are

● 	to <u>recognize</u> that you are a spiritual being, and

● 	to <u>accept</u> that you are a spiritual being.

Then you will be in a position to deal with your spirituality just as you deal with the growth and development of your finances, relationships, and career. Spirituality is an important part of your life. It requires your understanding and your attention. You can keep it in perspective and keep it growing in a way which is balanced with your other Areas of Life.

Under no circumstances should you feel guilty about your spirituality. If you exercise your instincts, develop your intuition and look into different doctrines, you will find the set of beliefs that brings you both peace of mind and a sense of inner peace for that period in your life. When that happens, you will experience the sense of grounding that a system of beliefs and principles provides all happy people.

Step 2: How to Create MY SPIRITUAL PLAN

You should now have an accurate perspective on spirituality. It is something that everyone has within. It is your faith, the beliefs that you hold in the face of otherwise unexplained happenings. It is how you see yourself in the context of the universe in which you exist. It is enveloped by the entire system of beliefs and principles by which you live. To be happy and fulfilled, you need to understand, to accept and to nurture this intuitive side of your life.

Every organized religion provides a recipe for your spirituality, although each church takes a slightly different approach in terms of beliefs, rituals, and requirements. You should experiment. Compare the primary tenets of several churches and evaluate them with respect to your own system of beliefs and principles.

If you find one with which you're compatible, then adopt it as the cornerstone of your spiritual life. If you can't find an existing organization which fits you, then you're on your own. Exercise your instincts just as you exercise your body, your mind and your emotions.

But in either case, you need to keep in mind the perspective you have just read as you

1   Make a commitment to understand your spirituality instead of trying to hide it or pretend it doesn't exist.

2   Set GOALS for the future that will foster your spiritual growth so that you can experience inner peace.

3   Plan ACTIONS that will develop your intuitive side of life so that you can enjoy the sense of grounding that accompanies a comfortable system of beliefs and principles.

Remember, people who are wise give the growth and development of their spiritual life a full 20% of their time and energy. How does your allocation measure up? Have you checked KEEPER #5—MY WHEEL OF BALANCE lately?

The first thing to do in creating KEEPER #7B—MY SPIRITUAL PLAN is to write down your spiritual GOAL. As before, it's supposed to support your PURPOSE. You may already have recorded your spiritual goal on KEEPER #6—MY PURPOSE WORKSHEET.

If you have, all you need to do is transcribe it. If not, right now, while you are focused on the Spiritual Area of Life set a target for yourself. Make yourself decide what you will do to nurture the growth and development of the intuitive side of your life. Be sure your GOAL supports your PURPOSE. Make sure it is reachable. At this point, you don't have to know how to achieve it, but it should be what you want to shoot for in the foreseeable future.

For example, I transcribed my Spiritual GOAL which supports my PURPOSE.

PURPOSE: *Using my analytical skills and objective perspective on life, I will be a counselor and coach to my clients, students, family and friends, while being guided by a strong sense of service and integrity.*

SPIRITUAL GOAL: *Become a "wise" person who has life in perspective and can advise others how to make progress toward their desired objectives.*

When I created this GOAL, I didn't have a clue how I was going to get there. But, I knew that if I could achieve it, I would be prepared spiritually TO BE who my PURPOSE says I AM.

> "Begin to weave & God
> will give you the thread."
> —German Proverb

Now it's time to record your spiritual goal on MY SPIRITUAL PLAN. So, find that quiet spot again where you can meditate on this GOAL in order to come up with some alternate ACTION plans that will help you attain it. Don't forget to transcribe any of your spiritual ACTIONS from KEEPER #6—MY PURPOSE WORKSHEET. Those ACTIONS also will help you overcome your fears or better balance your life.

As you list each ACTION idea that comes to mind, write down any comments concerning the best time to implement it, just as you did with MY PHYSICAL PLAN. Recognizing the best set of conditions for trying something out allows you to look for and take advantage of opportunities as they arise.

> "Chance favors
> the prepared mind."
> —Louis Pasteur

MY SPIRITUAL PLAN

<u>GOAL</u> — (The target for my Spiritual life which will enable me to fulfill my PURPOSE):

_____

_____

_____

<u>ACTIONS</u> to consider   <u>Comments</u>

ACTIONS to consider	Comments
1.	
2.	
3.	
4.	
5.	
6.	
7.	
8.	
9.	
10.	
11.	
12.	
13.	
14.	

Congratulations! You have come another step closer in the process of taking control of your life. Let's revisit Table V to see where you stand.

TABLE V

How to Take Control of Your Life

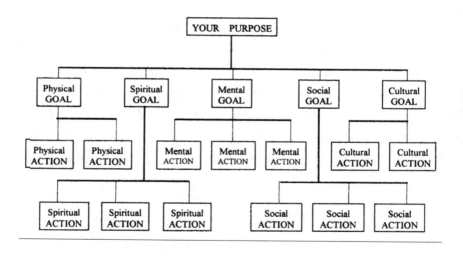

You have defined your PURPOSE and established your GOALS and ACTION plans for both the Physical and Spiritual Areas of Life. You are now in the driver's seat just about ready to "take the wheel." Three more Areas of Life to go and you will be on your way to a future of happiness, productivity and fulfillment.

How to Enjoy a Healthy Mental Life

Many people try to tolerate a stressful job situation. What they get instead is a major source of worry and concern.

Rationalizing work problems is easy and common. After all, the source of your paycheck may require a personal sacrifice occasionally. You may have to bring work home with you. You may feel a constant need to discuss your job with others just so you can keep it in perspective. And you may even find that your career is beginning to gobble up much more time and energy than it should. How much of this should a person tolerate?

Here are five questions to help you decide if occupational stress has become a problem for you.

1   Is it possible that my job is hindering my mental well-being?

2   Do my problems on the job carry over to other parts of my life?

3   Do I have nightmares about my workplace?

4   Do I engage in escape-type behavior (sleeping away the weekend or watching TV several hours a night) because of on-the-job stress?

5   Am I suffering from some stress-related illness such as high blood pressure, heart palpitations or high cholesterol?

If you replied "no" to four or five of these questions, consider yourself lucky. You've managed to avoid most of the perils of occupational stress. You'll probably find the following perspective on the subject to be only mildly interesting. Perhaps it will help you understand others and their stress levels. Zip through it, then get ready to create KEEPER #7C—MY MENTAL PLAN.

However, if your answer was "yes," "maybe" or perhaps "sometimes" to two or more of the questions, you need to think long and hard about what occupational stress is doing to your life. Here is a perspective that can help you put your mental life back on track.

Job Stress: Spotting and Beating This Occupational Hazard

Today's uncertain workplace often seems pitted with sink holes which can gobble you up at any moment. The biggest one is occupational stress. It results from a mismatch between your personality and the work environment.

Occupational stress has one result: It jangles your nerves. But it has two forms: Stress occurs when the incompatibility between your personality and your work environment causes excessive pressure on you. It also happens when you are at odds with your incompatible supervisor.

In either case, the longer you try to endure the situation the more likely it is to upset you and eventually lead to health problems. At its worst, stress can even shorten your life. You must watch for the telltale signs of this condition:

- headaches,

- short temper,

- fatigue,

- insomnia, and

- upset stomach.

And you must act decisively <u>before</u> stress takes control of your health and your life.

Remember, the underlying cause: A mismatch between your personality and your working environment. But, before looking closer at the nature and the cures for this problem, let's first define what stress really is. Acording to Dr. Hans Seyle, biological scientist and author of <u>Stress without Distress</u>, stress is "the nonspecific response of a body to any demand made upon it." In other words, anything to which we are exposed produces a need in us to adapt and re-establish normalcy.

A certain amount of stress is healthy. It motivates us to make decisions and achieve goals. In that way, stress helps people lead productive lives.

It is also a very personal experience. What is stress for me may bore you into yawning fits. Even if we both are stressed by the same thing, our stress levels may be different. If there is a looming deadline on an important project, one of us may be stressed to the point of paralysis. The other one of us might zip right through whatever needs to be done.

Even so, some kinds of stress are common in almost every workplace. These stresses are the result of mismatches between your personality and

1) Your job (the role you're required to play)

or

2) Your supervisor's personality.

Psychologists call this the Person-Environment Fit Model of Stress. It's shown as a triangle like this:

CHART 2

YOUR PERSONALITY

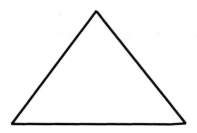

YOUR SUPERVISOR'S PERSONALITY

YOUR JOB ROLE

Obviously, it's impossible for everyone to get along well with everyone else. The fact that two people work for the same organization is no guarantee they'll be compatible. As with any relationship, it depends on how the personalities mesh in terms of traits and interests and beliefs and principles.

For example, let's suppose a person who works under you has a greater need for power than you do. Let's say this person puts a higher value on money and a lower value on truth than you do. Taking it a step further, this person could be willing to stab you in the back just to get your job. Now that's stress— big time!

Similarly, you and your job responsibilities may be a bad match. If you are an analytical, reflective person who is introverted, the job of selling boats or cars would probably drive you nuts. That kind of job role requires you to be a creative and aggressive extrovert who can relate superficially and simply. The pressure of being required to behave like a salesperson and not be yourself is going to have you battling between who you are and who you aren't every moment you're on that job.

Several stressors are very common in the workplace. They include:

- having too much to do,

- having too many deadlines,

- getting promoted too quickly or too slowly, and

- not being trained properly.

In the final analysis, however, all these problems can be traced to your being incompatible with either your superior or your job. This doesn't mean that you should always avoid overextending yourself or that backlogs of work and project deadlines are naturally bad for you. Sometimes such stresses can and do motivate people and beef up their productivity.

But too much is too much! When the stresses become so intense they're causing you harm, it's time to take a long look at your job situation. Persistent distress over a period can and likely will make you sick. Unfortunately, many people don't know or admit they are overstressed until they become chronically ill.

WHAT CAN YOU DO TO PROTECT YOUR MENTAL HEALTH?

In fact, there's only one cure for this common occupational problem: CHANGE. But before you can prescribe the specific cure, you have to diagnose the illness. You must identify the mismatch as being between either:

1) you and your boss,

or

2) you and your job role.

If the problem is your boss, there's not much you can do to repair the problem. Your boss is whomever he or she is. And, you are whomever you are. Oh, you can try a new attitude for a while, but that's a temporary fix at best. Your personality is well established and it just happens to be incompatible with your boss' personality. Do you think your boss is about to leave the organization? That would just be a stroke of pure luck.

You also can't rely on the nature of your job role changing in a way that will relieve your stress. At best, you may be able to make minor improvements to give yourself some breathing room.

In either case, your optimal strategy is to start looking for other opportunities. Of course, you'd be just plain lucky if you could advance your career when you are faced with either a boss or a job that's doing damage to you. Depending on your education, age, experience, the size of your organization, and the degree of specialty in your field, you should probably consider:

- a move within the organization (probably lateral),

- a move to another organization (possibly less pay),

- a career change (possibly an entry level position).

The important thing to remember is the need to initiate CHANGE! Right now you are endangering your well-being. If you continue to tolerate this situation, you could be chronically damaging your health.

> "Even if you're on the right track,
> you'll get run over
> if you just sit there."
> —Will Rogers

Occupational stress is an extremely common syndrome among the personnel employed in the workplace. Unfortunately, too many go on tolerating this dangerous condition. If you are suffering from this tendency, you are jeopardizing your mental well being.

Look for the forerunners of stress (too much to do, too little time, don't know how to do it). Life is too short to put up with a mismatch in your workplace. You are the only one concerned enough to do something about it. Only you can decide what changes are most likely to produce positive results. Remember, it's never too late to take action!

Step 3: How to Create MY MENTAL PLAN

You can help pull yourself out of job stress and feed your mind some good nourishment as well if you prepare a plan that will invigorate your mind.

As you prepare to record your mental goals and actions on KEEPER #7C—MY MENTAL PLAN, you should focus on the enjoyable things that exercise your mind in a positive way. What are the things that get the neurons in your brain all fired up? A great novel, a challenging debate, a difficult crossword puzzle, an afternoon in the library, a session on the Net? And what shuts down your grey matter faster than flipping a switch: A boring lecture, a B-film, a poorly written recipe or instruction booklet, a one-sided ball game?

You need to distinguish between these positive and negative mental influences. When you do start to create MY MENTAL PLAN, you'll identify ways to spark your imagination. You will begin to do things that will make your mind much more active. You'll identify learning goals and actions that will excite you. And, as you begin working on KEEPER #7C, don't forget the importance to your mental health of dealing with occupational stress.

If job-related problems have begun to preoccupy your mind both day and night, the mental stress may already be interfering with the rest of your life: relationships, physical conditioning and personal growth. This is bad for you and you know it. Be sure to incorporate some appropriate changes into MY MENTAL PLAN to get rid of these stress symptoms.

Now that you're focused on the mental side on your life, the best way to come up with a mental goal is to meditate on your PURPOSE. Think about your life's work and <u>what</u> you can do from an educational standpoint. These thoughts will help ensure that you become WHO YOU ARE somewhere down the road. Just be sure to emphasize things that will enhance your mental health. And remember, these goals need to be reachable for you sometime in the future.

> "No one knows what he can do until he tries."
> —Publilius Syrus

Take another look at Table V so you can see where you are in the overall process. Remember, you have your Physical and Spiritual Plans already constructed and your Social and Cultural Plans still to create.

TABLE V

How to Take Control of Your Life

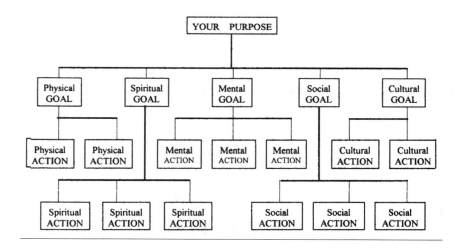

Here's how this works for me. To support my PURPOSE (*using my analytical skills and objective perspective on life, I will be a counselor and coach to my clients, students, family and friends, while being guided by a strong sense of service and integrity*), I set the following Mental GOAL for myself:

"Get to know myself objectively in terms of my traits, beliefs and principles. I must also understand the impact of other people's behavior on me, and the impact of changes occurring in society on me."

You can see why this is a mental goal. It involves the acquisition of knowledge (mental) and it explains <u>what</u> I'm going to do (a goal). It also supports my PURPOSE since achieving this GOAL will better prepare me to serve others in the role of a coach and counselor. It doesn't, however, address <u>how</u> I'm going to do it—those are the ACTIONS that come next.

You know the routine. Find a quiet spot and meditate just like you did on your other GOALS. Come up with some ACTIONS to support that goal. Record your ideas on KEEPER #7C—MY MENTAL PLAN. Don't forget to include any of your good Mental ideas already residing on KEEPER #6. Then, indicate in the "Comments" column anything that will jog your memory later about the timing or conditions that would favor using that ACTION.

"Man's mind,
once stretched by a new idea,
never regains its original dimension."

—Oliver Wendell Holmes

MY MENTAL PLAN

<u>GOAL</u> — (The target for my Mental life which will enable me to fulfill my PURPOSE):

_____

_____

_____

ACTIONS to consider	Comments
1.	
2.	
3.	
4.	
5.	
6.	
7.	
8.	
9.	
10.	
11.	
12.	
13.	
14.	

When you complete MY MENTAL PLAN, take a break. You now have a plan for three of the five Areas of Life. These are the three areas: Physical, Spiritual and Mental that are probably underweight on your Wheel of Balance. By focusing on these first, you have ensured that your life will be more balanced in the future. You have identified a GOAL and ACTION plan for each of these areas that will help you to experience your PURPOSE. Your fulfillment of realizing your life's work is another step closer.

But don't rest for too long. You still have two more Areas of Life to put into perspective. Not until you define your Social and Cultural GOALS and ACTIONS will you have a cohesive road map to your future. Only then will you be in the driver's seat with your hands on the wheel.

> "True happiness consists not in the multitude of friends, but in the worth and choice."
> —Ben Jonson

SECTION 8D

How to Enjoy a Happy Social Life

Lots of people are making themselves miserable by passively allowing someone they don't really like or enjoy into their lives. You need people in your life who are compatible with you, people who complement what you are like and share your beliefs and principles.

To have a happy social life, you must understand what forms the foundation for a genuinely compatible relationship—then act on it. To allow people you don't enjoy to remain a part of your social life is only going to put you in an ugly mood. A mood which is going to spill over to people you truly do care about.

It's time to look at yourself again. Are you a nervous wreck because you are trying to include in your life people with whom you just don't get along? Here are five questions to help you decide if you understand the foundation for compatibility between people:

1   Do I find emotional stability in my relationships?

2   Do my relationships energize me in a positive way?

3   Do I know when my personality meshes with others?

4   Are my friends and relatives a source of support and happiness to me?

5   Am I "myself" around my friends?

If you can honestly answer "yes" to four or five of these questions, your social life is already the backbone of your emotional strength. The following perspective on relationships will probably be of marginal interest to you. Zip through it, then dig into KEEPER #7D—MY SOCIAL PLAN.

However, if two or more of your responses were "no" or "maybe" or "sometimes," you need to review what a compatible relationship really is. For you, MY SOCIAL PLAN should include some new opportunities for you to express your love and to enjoy a happier social life in the future.

Relationships: Finding and Hanging onto "Good People" in Your Life

You can't go off and live by yourself. You need to be in touch with other people so you can grow emotionally and flourish as a human being.

> "When one helps another,
> both are strong."
> —German Proverb

People with truly compatible friends have discovered something invaluable: friends and other important relationships form the emotional foundation of their lives. If you are compatible with someone else, contact with them energizes you, stimulates you, makes you feel that you're growing. Real friends support each other in all experiences, both happy and sad.

Psychologists have known for years that everyone is a bit different from everyone else. Some people can get along with almost anyone while there are those who put people on edge just by being around. Most people, of course, are a blend of the two—getting along with some but not with others.

The psychologists have even developed tests such as the Personality Analysis System contained on the computer disk accompanying this book to analyze and describe individual personalities. Psychologists, however, have not been as successful at figuring out how two or more people will get along.

RESOURCE BOX

One psychological test that has been developed for testing the compatibility of relationships is called FIRO which stands for Fundamental Interpersonal Relations Orientation. It is available through the Consulting Psychologists Press to qualified practitioners.

This means you're pretty much on your own when it comes to finding compatible friends, people who complement your traits and share your beliefs.

Fortunately, compatible friends are not that hard to find if you know what you're looking for. People move around so easily that you literally meet thousands of potential friends during your lifetime.

Almost every day you have the opportunity to go through the process of making acquaintances and finding a kindred spirit.

The question is, how good are you at identifying compatible relationships? One way to grade yourself is to ask, "If my life hit a crisis, who would I turn to?" If you can't come up with more than a name or two, you should start putting time into creating and preserving good relationships.

Yes, finding and maintaining good relationships can be time consuming—particularly when you're just using the trial and error method. If the divorce rate is any indication, many people are using that approach not only when selecting friends but also when choosing a spouse.

SOME GUIDELINES FOR FINDING RELATIONSHIPS THAT WORK

First, check your own attitude about what you think makes people compatible. You may have been misdirecting yourself.

For example, don't look for common interests as the <u>fundamental</u> basis for friendship. Finding people to go bowling or golfing with is not a path to finding a deep relationship. It's only a road to finding people who share your kind of recreation and want to enjoy a good time, nothing more.

On a level just as superficial, searching for love among the best-looking specimens of the opposite sex may provide some good eye candy for a little while. But, it's a foolish way to find the person best for your heart.

Instead of using the "skin-deep approach," search for people you will really treasure. Those are the people

- whose strengths and limitations complement your own,

- whose beliefs you share, and

- whose principles are compatible with your own.

Of course, this assumes that you know who you are. Any doubts? Sneak a peek back at KEEPER #1—MY RESOURCES. You created this summary of your traits (strengths and limitations), beliefs and principles. Remember? Now is a good time to look it over again.

Next, consider the other person's principles relative to what is most important to you. Examining another's principles is an excellent way of measuring whether they are the kind of person you want in your life. Try to determine how important the following principles are to them:

- Integrity

- Love

- Wisdom

- Thrift

- Moderation

If someone values two or more of these principles far differently than you do, the two of you are unlike enough fundamentally to blow a hole in any kind of deep relationship. Someone who values these elements to the same extent you do is a good prospect for being compatible—a person you will want to spend quality time with.

Next think about traits. Since people behave in different ways, their personalities can either mesh or clash. Consider prospective friends from the standpoint of such traits as

- control and the exercise of power,

- goal-setting and achievement,

- the need to belong, and

- the expression of and need for affection.

For example, if two individuals both crave power and control, they are likely to end in a power struggle, not a relationship. Dominance in one person and submission in the other is a much more compatible combination. Similarly, two people driven to achieve will likely end up competing with (rather than complementing) each other. And, if one person has a much stronger need for affection than the other person has for giving it, well, there's a relationship headed nowhere.

That's why it's very important to learn whether someone else's traits complement yours. If they do, then, and ONLY THEN, should you begin encouraging interactions based on common interests and activities. Just remember, two people can reconcile many seemingly conflicting interests if their traits, principles, and beliefs are in alignment.

For example, a person who wants to have enough money to bail out of the work force at an early age could be compatible with someone who wants to travel the world. But, then again, two people who differ widely on how much money to give to those less fortunate would likely clash because their principles are so opposite.

True, this approach to screening potential relationships can gobble up some time. It requires you to get to know someone well enough to understand his or her traits, principles and beliefs. It's much easier to decide you're compatible with someone based on whether they look sexy, have a lot of money or like long walks as much as you do. None of these factors has much to do with what someone is really like as a person.

More and more people seem to resort to astrology to check for the compatibility of their "signs." Some consult biorhythms to see if their cycles are compatible before pursuing a relationship. Bunk. Doesn't a method based on some understanding of what people believe, what principles guide them and how they behave, make a lot more sense?

Look, you don't have to make looking for compatible people play like a military drill. And you don't want to be microscopically examining others for flaws and quirks every time you're with them.

You can still be enjoyable to be around, even while you're scanning others to see if they might be compatible with you. Just don't force it. Let the traits, beliefs and principles of others display themselves naturally as the relationship develops. You'll know soon enough whether someone will be a compatible long-term friend, or nothing more than a bowling buddy.

Just as incompatible relationships are emotionally chaotic and stressful, compatible friendships and positive intimate relationships are emotionally stabilizing. They should provide you with security and help you to pursue your life's ambitions. They should be a source of energy and help you overcome unwanted stress. They should make your life easier and help you to better understand yourself.

True fulfillment is not possible without a few significant relationships. It's vitally important for you to have in your life compatible relationships in which you're committed. Although our culture stresses independence, too much can lead to isolation. You must overcome the tendency to leave friends behind in favor of a search for more money, success, or fame. That is NOT a happy, healthy or wise way to live.

As you prepare KEEPER #7D—MY SOCIAL PLAN, remember that the cornerstones of good relationships are compatible personalities. Finding good friends, people who support each other in good times and bad, is well worth the time it takes. Your life will be far richer, far more interesting, far more worthwhile, if you can identify the people who can help form the emotional foundation of your life.

PAYOFF BOX

Don't deprive yourself. Pick up the phone and call someone from your past with whom you know you're compatible. Good relationships are worth the effort.

are emotionally stabilizing. They should provide you with security and help you to pursue your life's ambitions. They should be a source of energy and help you overcome unwanted stress. They should make your life easier and help you to better understand yourself.

True fulfillment is not possible without a few significant relationships. It's vitally important for you to have in your life compatible relationships in which you're committed. Although our culture stresses independence, too much can lead to isolation. You must overcome the tendency to leave friends behind in favor of a search for more money, success, or fame. That is NOT a happy, healthy or wise way to live.

As you prepare KEEPER #7D—MY SOCIAL PLAN, remember that the cornerstones of good relationships are compatible personalities. Finding good friends, people who support each other in good times and bad, is well worth the time it takes. Your life will be far richer, far more interesting, far more worthwhile, if you can identify the people who can help form the emotional foundation of your life.

PAYOFF BOX

Don't deprive yourself. Pick up the phone and call someone from your past with whom you know you're compatible. Good relationships are worth the effort.

● Think about the social aspects of your life that you enjoy and are good for you. That way your Social GOAL and ACTIONS will involve the positive ones (dating, family gatherings and parties) and skip the unhappy ones (difficult people, peer pressure and control freaks).

● Keep in mind the indispensable need for compatible relationships in your life to provide you with emotional support and stability.

● Review KEEPER #6—MY PURPOSE WORKSHEET to make sure that you include in MY SOCIAL PLAN any of those good ideas that will help you overcome your fears or balance your life so you can remove these obstacles forever.

● Meditate on your PURPOSE to define your Social GOAL—your target for interacting with others five or ten or 20 years down the road that will enable you to be who your PURPOSE says you are.

● Meditate on your Social GOAL to come up with possible ACTION plans for meeting people which will help you achieve that GOAL.

● Include in MY SOCIAL PLAN the best time or conditions for putting each of your possible ACTION plans into, well, action.

For example, based on my PURPOSE,

"Using my analytical skills and objective perspective on life, I will be a counselor and coach to my clients, students, family and friends, while being guided by a strong sense of service and integrity,"

I identified the following GOAL and ACTIONS on my KEEPER #7D—MY SOCIAL PLAN. Since I prepared this Plan at a time when our circle of friends was already a positive influence in our lives, you will notice that the primary emphasis dealt with our family relationships.

After reviewing my entries, follow the procedure outlined above and create your own KEEPER #7D—MY SOCIAL PLAN. It won't be long before you discover the happiness of an emotionally stable social life in which your relationships complement and complete you.

Don't forget to focus on compatible friendships. Reach out to those who share your beliefs and complement your traits and principles. You will find that true friends anticipate each other's needs, help each other realize their dreams and support each other through the rough times. When you plan interactions with compatible friends and relatives, you create a happy social life.

> # "A friend
> # is a gift
> # you give yourself."
>
> # —Robert Louis Stevenson

MY SOCIAL PLAN

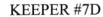

GOAL — (The target for my Social life which will enable me to fulfill my PURPOSE):

<u>Provide a secure and stable home for my family so that our children will feel free to "return" while getting oriented into the cultural worlds of higher education and work.</u>

ACTIONS to consider   Comments

ACTIONS to consider	Comments
1. Support wife's childrearing ideas	Reinforce her decisions
2. Encourage kid's strengths	Whenever observed
3. Listen to kids	When <u>they</u> want to talk
4. Maintain home and grounds	Encourage kids to help
5. Plan family outings	Weekly
6. Attend kid's functions	Sports and school
7.	
8.	
9.	
10.	
11.	
12.	

MY SOCIAL PLAN

<u>GOAL</u> — (The target for my Social life which will enable me to fulfill my PURPOSE):

_____

_____

_____

<u>ACTIONS to consider</u>   <u>Comments</u>

ACTIONS to consider	Comments
1.	
2.	
3.	
4.	
5.	
6.	
7.	
8.	
9.	
10.	
11.	
12.	
13.	
14.	

You have now assembled four-fifths of your Plan for the future—a future in which you are in control. You have designed ACTION plans that will exercise your body, mind, emotions and instincts. Included in your Plan are some ideas that will challenge your fears and others that will simplify your life. A future of happiness, good health, wealth and wisdom is practically yours—it's right around the next bend in the road.

You have shown tremendous patience in waiting until last to craft your Cultural Plan. This is the one that most people think about first, the one where you get to show off your marketable skills. Included in your Cultural Plan will be your moneymaking ideas, your career plans and your expressions of materialism.

By focusing on the other Areas of Life first, you can be assured that your natural gifts—body, mind, emotions and instincts—will be properly cared for. Now it's time to put the Cultural Area of Life into perspective and make sure that your future includes the wealth that you want.

> "I am only one;
> but still I am one.
> I cannot do everything,
> but still I can do something;
> I will not refuse to do
> the something I can do."
> —Helen Keller

How to Enjoy a Wealthy Cultural Life

People tend to fall into two major cultural traps. The first concerns career and the second involves money. Both have a great deal to do with your status in the eyes of others. Why? Because cultural activities involve showing off symbols of success (dollars, possessions, power and achievement). These symbols effect your potential for financial independence and also your happiness, health and wisdom.

Bad things happen when people pursue careers for the WRONG reasons:

- continuing the family business,

- the money is good,

- it sounds prestigious,

- others find it interesting, or

- can't think of anything else to do.

The usual sequence of events goes something like this. After investing significant time and energy on education and training, people enter the workplace feeling like fish out of water. They find themselves playing a role they don't enjoy. They become stressed and dissatisfied. They begin to dislike themselves and the fallout of some bad career decision carries over into the other areas of their lives.

Here are five short questions to help you decide if you're having this problem.

1   Do I enjoy my career?

2   Did I choose the right career for me?

3   Did I consider my personality when I selected my career?

4   Did I consider the job "role" that I would be expected to play?

5   Does my career reinforce my self-esteem?

If you voiced a resounding "yes" to four or five of these questions, you're in good shape. You have found a compatible career situation in which you'll probably be productive, happy and successful. The following perspective on careers will only serve to confirm the wisdom of your choice.

However, two or more negative or unsure answers mean you'll get a lot out of reading about career decision-making before completing KEEPER 7E—MY CULTURAL PLAN. Your career should be rewarding and fulfilling, not just a source of income.

Careers: Identifying the "Right Job" for You

Of the major life choices that you make, your career is one of the most important. It has a way of <u>becoming</u> you. And, you have to invest a great deal of time into it. Counting lunch breaks, preparation time and commuting, your work probably consumes 12 hours of your day and sometimes more.

In short, your job swallows half of each day and as much as

three-fourths of all the time you're awake. Actually, it's more. Even when you're not "on the clock," it can be hard to just flip a switch and stop thinking about work. In your off-hours, you probably find yourself talking-out work problems with family or friends and evaluating possible career moves.

In fact, work situations, conditions and people may even invade your dreams at night. Making a poor career decision is something you have to live with literally day and night.

So, what standards should you use in making your career decision? There is no easy answer. Some people know at an early age what they want to do "when I grow up." Others gravitate toward a career which uses their favorite subject in school or college. Still others seek professional help in finding a career direction based on an analysis of their interests. For some, money is a primary concern. But money should be only one factor.

More importantly, your career may dominate your lifestyle off the job: the way you spend your time and the friends you associate with. Let's face it! Your career is a major role that you act out in life.

> "All the world's a stage
> and all the men and women
> merely players."
> —Shakespeare

That's right. Being a brain surgeon or a teacher or a bricklayer requires playing a specific role. One part of being successful at work is to properly portray the image that society attaches to that profession or career or job.

The fact that your boss gives you a good performance review further verifies the fact that you are "performing" a role when you do your job. Good performances are "applauded" with pay increases and promotions; poor ones do not get calls for an "encore."

PERSONAL RECOGNITION ACCOMPANIES A CAREER

There is more than one reason why the job role you "play" *becomes* such an enormous part of who you are.

First, people identify you with your career role and expect you to behave consistently with the public image that it brings to mind. For example, a successful doctor is expected to be analytical, methodical, rational, friendly, helpful, persuasive, insightful, understanding, and instructive.

So, if your major characteristics are being persistent, practical, stable, shy, reliable, impulsive, conscientious, efficient, and obedient, it would be very difficult for you to "play the role" of a doctor. However, with these traits, you might enjoy very much driving a truck for a living. This comparison highlights the contrast in personality which society underline expects from individuals in different professional roles.

Secondly, the amount of time you devote to playing your work role makes it difficult for you to be a different kind of person when you are "offstage" in your personal life. Your satisfaction, happiness, and comfort depend upon your ability to find a role or roles which fit you and your personality. If you find yourself in a job role which fits your personality like a badly-made suit, what you'll get is a strong dose of stress. This comes from trying to cope with a bad situation instead of the fulfillment of being in a career that's natural for you.

RESOURCE BOX

The importance of personality in career success and enjoyment is recognized and well documented. John L. Holland's <u>Making Vocational Choices: A Theory of Careers</u> defines six clusters of personality traits into which all people can be categorized and all work situations can be classified. The exercise of choosing a career becomes a two-step process of (1) identifying your major personality type, and (2) deciding which work roles reward you for expressing your traits, interests, principles and beliefs.

Whether you're making your first career choice or a subsequent one, you need to be acutely aware of the importance of the compatibility between your personality and your work role.

EXAMPLES OF CAREER MATCHES AND MISMATCHES

I made a huge mistake early on, and I ended up with a personality mismatch which clanged in my head every day I was on the job. When I was in my twenties, I decided to open my own consulting business. I had the education, the experience, the drive and the commitment to succeed. The trouble was, I was miserable from the first day I opened the doors. I hadn't anticipated how I would feel when I was trying to sell people on using my services.

The problem was this: I'm an introspective person. I like to think and to approach people in a low-key and cautious manner. Unfortunately, my prospective clients were expecting an entirely different kind of "salesman-type" person. They expected someone who was extremely comfortable around people, who would push them hard to use my services. They actually <u>liked</u> consultants using the hard sell on them. I wasn't that kind of person and never will be. I could see that I wasn't pulling in enough business. I also could see that, considering my personality and my clients' expectations, my future as an independent consultant was bleak.

I was fighting myself and fighting myself hard. I suffered from several health problems and eventually—no surprise here—had to close that business. If I'd only understood myself well enough to grasp what a mismatch I was going to create, I could have completely avoided that business and medical disaster.

Someone else with a different personality and the same knowledge and skill might have succeeded brilliantly where I failed so miserably. That's life—we learn from our mistakes. The fact is that we are all suited to doing some things and not others. To a large extent, it depends on our traits, interests, principles and beliefs.

Another way to think about this point is to try to answer the following question: What do a social science teacher, a parole officer, a TV repair person and a certified public accountant have in common? No, this is not a riddle. I'm serious. What do they have in common?

Obviously, these professions are very different in terms of their educational requirements, earnings expectations, and field of interest. However, they share the common thread of requiring people who hold these jobs to enjoy:

1   frequently interacting with others,

2   using diagnostic methods to get information, and

3   routinely keeping records.

People who enjoy this balance of social interaction, intellectual stimulation, and routine paperwork share many personality characteristics. In fact, if you're looking for happiness, personality is probably <u>more important</u> than either education or earnings potential when it comes to career choice.

When your work role is compatible with your personality, you will greatly increase your chances of being productive, being successful, and experiencing a sense of fulfillment in your work. Why? Because you'll find your job to be natural, easy and rewarding.

If you find yourself in a job role that doesn't feel right, it probably isn't right for you. Don't despair. It's not too late to fix your problem. In our society, there is terrific geographic and occupational mobility.

You should never trap yourself into a dissatisfying, unrewarding, or stressful work situation for more than a brief period. When you are in an incompatible work situation, you need to make a change. Since you can't significantly change who you are, it's necessary to change your job or even your career (the role that you play more than half of each day).

Furthermore, when making future career choices, you must remember that <u>the most important</u> part of the decision is finding a work environment that matches your personality. That match, more than any other factor, will determine your future happiness and success.

> "Choose a job you love,
> and you will never
> have to work
> a day in your life."
> —Chinese Proverb

The second most common cultural problem also concerns money. The usual scenario is that people don't have enough, even when they have a "good job" and can make "good money." Insecurity creeps into the picture, stress over financial matters mounts and the resulting feelings spill over into other Areas of Life. Does this picture resemble your financial situation?

Try answering the following five questions:

1   Do I earn enough money?

2   Can I afford to buy everything I want?

3   Can I save more money?

4   Will I be able to retire early?

5   Will I ever achieve financial independence?

If you answered "yes" to four or five of these questions, congratulations! You have managed to avoid the common financial hazard that stops so many from taking control of their lives. A quick pass through the following discussion on "money" will suffice. You'll probably pick up a tip or two in the process to secure your future wealth.

However, if you found yourself wavering or responding "no" to two or more of these questions, you'll benefit greatly from the following perspective. It holds the secrets to your future financial peace of mind.

Money: Making and Keeping Enough Legally to be Set Financially

Conventional wisdom says that the only ways to become financially independent are to be born rich, inherit a large sum at an early age or win the lottery. The rest of us, so this wisdom goes, must all work 40 years to support our desired standard of living. We must also make sure we have enough money for a decent retirement.

That's ridiculous! It's still possible in this country to start with no financial resources. It is possible to earn enough money to support a family. It's also possible to accumulate enough money to become financially independent in time to enjoy it. And you can achieve all three of these ends by doing work which is legal, moral and honest.

Admittedly, it takes a little effort. You need some self-discipline, and you have to pay strict attention to some basic financial concepts. You see, the biggest problem that we face in achieving financial independence isn't earning enough money. We all see plenty of money pass through our hands. The problem is **holding on to what we make.**

The following six financial ideas will show you how to overcome the biggest temptations to spend your hard-earned money. By sticking fast to these principles, you will hold on to a significant percentage of your earnings each year. You will accumulate wealth slowly and steadily. If you are diligent and get a good head start, you can achieve financial independence while you're still young enough to enjoy it.

IDEA 1: SAVE

You've heard this one before . . . But saving is one of those ideas that is much easier to talk about than to do. Pressures abound to spend, but there aren't many incentives to nudge you into socking money away. Even the government contributes to the problem by taxing the interest we earn on our savings.

How about saving to buy a home? Even that popular notion has lost its punch. Renting looks like a good option in many areas of the country. And home prices don't seem to jump up in value the way they used to. In some areas, the cost is so prohibitive that the "American Dream" has drastically changed. It has become a search to find someone who will give you the down payment on your house so you can afford to borrow the remainder.

Saving to send children to college used to be in vogue. But, with tuition costs soaring, many families feel that putting together the money themselves is a fantasy. Instead, they hope their children will somehow snag scholarships or work their way through college.

Certainly we all still need to save for retirement. Here the government has given us some sweetener for our savings, including the added tax incentive provided for Individual Retirement Accounts, Roth IRA's, employer supported 401(K) Plans, and Keogh Plans for the self-employed.

Unfortunately, all too many people don't take advantage of these highly useful ways to make retirement savings grow. Instead, these same people continue to rely on the promise of Social Security retirement benefits and, if they're lucky, an employer's pension plan. Well, don't hold your breath waiting for that pension. The U.S. Labor Department reports that nearly six out of ten workers in the private sector reach age 65 with absolutely no pension at all.

In short, you have to rely on yourself. Hoping other people will bail you out will never lead to financial independence. The best method is to save, save, save. How? Pay yourself first! Take 10%, 20% or even 25% right off the top of your paycheck and put it into your savings account or your mutual fund account. Start on your next payday and keep doing it. It's one habit you will never regret.

Let's look at some numbers to see what this practice can do for your long-range financial picture. If you earn $50,000/year for 20 years, that's one million dollars that will be paid to you, before taxes. If you save 25% of each paycheck, that's $250,000 in the bank!

Actually, adjusted for interest earned and compounded along the way, it's significantly <u>more</u> than that. But, at 10% interest, that $250,000 is equivalent to a lifetime income of $25,000 per year. Can you live on that? Many people can and do!

IDEA 2: BUY ONLY WHAT YOU <u>NEED</u>

The money you spend should be a direct reflection of your needs. There is no point in trying to imitate or compete with what other people are buying or consuming. You'll spend a lot more than you need or want to.

Here's the sad part: The more you spend on unnecessary things, the more time you must spend <u>working</u> to make sure you have a decent retirement. Wouldn't you rather retire at 55? At 65? Some people can't afford to retire and must work well into their seventies. Don't let that be you.

Winners in the game of life are not the people who "own the most toys when they die." Owning a depreciating boat which is used only one or two weeks a year may temporarily make you a big shot in the neighborhood. But, it also means you have to work extra months or even years to accumulate the money you need to indulge this whim or pay off the loan.

ASK YOURSELF BEFORE BUYING: *"How much more time will this purchase keep me chained to the work force?"*

Using that yardstick, many potential purchases will seem silly or self-indulgent. If something you want to buy is going to satisfy only your need for status, why spend the cash? Ultimately, your status isn't measured by how much you own. Your success in life is determined by the extent to which you achieve personal fulfillment and make a contribution to the lives of others. That's why you have spent time creating KEEPER #6—MY PURPOSE WORKSHEET.

IDEA 3: WATCH TV COMMERCIALS AND READ THE NEWSPAPER FOR INFORMATION ONLY

One of the biggest traps confronting people is paying too much attention to commercial advertisements. True, entertainment and news reports help us to balance our lives. But, if you don't tune out the commercials which accompany them, you may end up buying things you don't need for reasons which are not important. Do you need that new car because a sexy lady in a bikini is leaning against it? Do you really need to buy potato chips because some cute cartoon character says you should?

Our capitalist economy is driven by consumption. Not surprisingly, there are daily pressures on us to spend, spend, spend. It used to be the door-to-door encyclopedia salesman who preyed on the weak, the uninitiated, the uninformed and persuaded them to part with their money.

Today it's the advertising agencies who go well beyond the limits of mere information to deliberately manipulate. Television ads are not trying to fill a need. They're intended to create one. Why do we "need" soft drinks when water is so plentiful and essentially free? We don't really need them, of course. Even so, commercial television messages have us believing that we not only need soft drinks but also can have the same "good life" people on the small screen are having if we buy specific brands.

ASK YOURSELF: *"Do I really need what I am thinking about buying?"*

The message should be clear: If you really need something, TV and newspaper ads can be a good source of what's available. But don't let yourself be victimized by the "needs" that advertisers try to create.

IDEA 4: LIVE WITHIN YOUR MEANS

If you're thinking of borrowing money to buy something, stop!

ASK YOURSELF: *"Will this purchase appreciate in value during the time that I own it?"*

Unless it will, don't <u>borrow</u> just so you can have it. Can't think of many examples of things that appreciate? That's because there aren't many. Housing is a good example of something that usually appreciates over the long term. Real estate in most areas shows an increase in value during an eight to ten year period. Plus, buying housing on credit can give you some terrific leverage and tax benefits that you just won't get otherwise.

Consumer credit, on the other hand, is a relatively new term. It has accompanied the rise of credit cards in the second half of the 20th century. If you stop and think about it, how can you justify buying something with money that you don't have? Has your need for immediate gratification become so overwhelming that you can't save and wait until you have the money to buy things?

Of course, it's very easy to get caught up in the borrowing habit. It's almost expected of you. Doesn't everyone do it? Sales pressures convince you that you <u>can</u> afford it on your wages or salary. After a while you don't even have to rationalize borrowing anymore. It almost becomes a reflex. The need for immediate gratification is a disease—a psychological disease just as powerful as any other addiction, whether it is nicotine, alcohol or some illegal drug.

Those who save and practice <u>delayed</u> gratification will be in a position to retire early. Those who borrow to consume are committing themselves to a life of slavery to the system, chained to the work force indefinitely. Remember that the U.S. Labor Department reports that nearly six of every ten workers in the private sector have no retirement funds at all when they reach age 65. Don't be one of them. Make your retirement the kind of life you really want it to be, not just what a meager Social Security check will allow.

IDEA 5: CONSERVE

The practice of questioning every dollar, every penny, you spend will go a long way toward conserving your earnings. Before handing over your credit card or hard-earned cash,

ASK YOURSELF:

- *"Am I really getting my money's worth here?"*

- *"Will this be on sale next week?"*

- *"Would I be better off saving this money?"* and

● *"Do I have a good reason to make this purchase?"*

The money you have is a result of your efforts; don't spend frivolously. Remember how much time and effort it took to accumulate that money. If you are thinking about buying something, write down a good reason for buying it. If you can't think of one, then don't buy it.

A good test to see if you are overindulging yourself is whether you sometimes feel guilty after spending money. If you do, chances are you aren't asking yourself the four questions above to decide whether or not a purchase is worthwhile.

On the other hand, if you are sometimes accused by your family or friends of being a "skinflint," that may be a good sign. Passing up a lot of chances to spend money can be a good thing. However, being stingy and cheap is one matter, being frugal is another. Frugality is a virtue.

For example, you are being frugal when you ride to work with a co-worker but you're being cheap if you never chip in for gas. Eating at inexpensive restaurants: FRUGAL. Not tipping: CHEAP. Buying good quality used furniture is an example of frugality. Doing all your shopping at garage sales is being cheap!

Experiment with the difference and settle upon a spending pattern and a savings rate that is comfortable for you.

IDEA 6: AT WORK, DELEGATE; AT HOME, DO IT YOURSELF

Conventional wisdom also says "if you want it done right, do it yourself." Most people obey this adage at work. There they want to impress a boss and get pay raises and promotions. Most people, however, disobey this advice in their personal lives. They pay others to handle such services as doing income taxes and repairing the car so, they say, they can enjoy their leisure time. These strategies are exactly the opposite of what you should be doing to maximize your long term financial well-being.

Here is the best strategy on the job. Once you have done something and done it well, try not to do it again. Assume the responsibility for it but delegate it to someone under you the next time it comes up. Learn to become an effective supervisor. Those who can supervise others increase their own earning power in the work force by showing they can control and direct large quantities of productive activity.

In your personal life, it's quite different. The more tasks you take care of yourself in your personal life, the more cash you will conserve. Of course, some jobs require special equipment—front-end alignments and emission controls, for example—and some require specialized education. Doctoring yourself when you're sick works only up to a point.

However, the more self-sufficient you are, the more money you will have in the future. Take advantage of do-it-yourself stores and free seminars. Trade your expertise with helpful neighbors and co-workers. Use diagnostic services, and any other lowcost alternatives to retail services. Remember, those who can handle their own chores save on cash-draining services.

❖

There's no shortage of advice on how to achieve financial independence. However, nothing is more straightforward than these six important concepts. Sticking to these basic but often-overlooked ideas will help you to exercise self-discipline. You'll hold on to your earnings and accumulate wealth slowly and steadily. If you start early and make even average earnings, you can expect to become financially independent and retire early. Think of this payoff the next time you are tempted to break one of the six ideas for taking control of your finances.

Step 5: How to Create MY CULTURAL PLAN

KEEPER #7E—MY CULTURAL PLAN has purposely been left until last. That's because you're not exercising one of your basic human faculties (body, mind, emotions and instincts) when you are operating in the cultural Area of Life. Here, you primarily exercise your marketable skills—those things you know how to do that allow you to manipulate and accumulate symbols of status like money, possessions, power and influence.

Consequently, the Cultural Area of Life is more of a secondary area. It is not <u>basic</u> to your existence. It is a product of humanity. There are four other Areas of Life that are <u>at least</u> as important and probably more important than the cultural area.

Even after reading this book, you may find this fact hard to believe. That's because there are just so many influences at work in society trying to make cultural interests the most significant aspect of your life. Think about all of your cultural roles and activities: working, shopping, investing, vacationing, housekeeping, watching TV, driving your car. What could be more important?

I hope by now you agree that your Physical, Mental, Social and Spiritual Areas of Life are at least AS important when it comes to achieving happiness, health, wealth and wisdom.

I'm not suggesting that you ignore your cultural life, but you need to make an extra and sustained effort to keep it in balance with the other areas. You remember KEEPER #5—MY WHEEL OF BALANCE. What is your cultural allocation of time relative to the 20% ideal? See what I mean? You must make a conscious effort to fight that tendency to let cultural things dominant your life.

That said, here's what you've been waiting for—a chance to document your cultural GOAL. On KEEPER #7E—MY CULTURAL PLAN, you should write down your cultural GOAL—where you want to go with your career and how much power, money and status you want to have.

This is just a target—<u>what</u> you hope to accomplish. It's not supposed to explain <u>how</u> you are going to get there. You should then brainstorm some ideas for achieving this objective as you begin writing down some alternative ACTION plans that you might try under ACTIONS to consider. You know the drill. It's the same process you have already completed for the other four Areas of Life.

When you are creating MY CULTURAL PLAN, be sure to include your good ideas contained on KEEPER #6—MY PURPOSE WORKSHEET. This valuable document will ensure that you incorporate into your cultural GOAL and ACTION plans ways of actively confronting your fears. You also need to incorporate ways of balancing your life by eliminating some of the complexities.

I am confident that you know by now how to create MY (AREA OF LIFE) PLAN. Just to remind you of the process, I meditated on my PURPOSE:

"Using my analytical skills and objective perspective on life, I will be a counselor and coach to my clients, students, family and friends, while being guided by a strong sense of service and integrity."

Out of this internal brainstorming came the following Cultural GOAL:

"Attain a position of financial independence so that I can 'retire' from the organizational world at an age young enough to pursue my primary mission in life."

I then went on to meditate on this GOAL until I could write down a whole list of ACTION plans on MY CULTURAL PLAN. I also indicated for each ACTION an appropriate time to put the plan into action.

So, go ahead, create KEEPER #7E so that you can gain the satisfaction of having a plan for each area of your life. This is your opportunity to introduce the balance that you want in your life, a future in which you are in control. You will no longer be looking to your boss, your friends, your relatives, your teachers nor your exercise coach for your happiness. You will just have to look in the mirror because YOU WILL BE IN CONTROL OF YOUR OWN DESTINY!

Think how you will feel after creating a set of targets you know you can reach, targets which will help you fulfill your purpose and reinforce your reason for being here. I'm excited for you, because I recall the surge of exhilaration I felt when I took control of my life. I remember thinking, "This is what it must feel like having a giant weight lifted from your shoulders. At last I am free to do what I want to do and be the person who I really am. I have just created a roadmap that shows me how to do it."

MY CULTURAL PLAN

GOAL — (The target for my Cultural life which will enable me to fulfill my PURPOSE):

_____

_____

_____

ACTIONS to consider	Comments
1.	
2.	
3.	
4.	
5.	
6.	
7.	
8.	
9.	
10.	
11.	
12.	
13.	
14.	

Now that you have completed your PLAN for each Area of Life, you should take an extra long break. Reflect on how far you've come on the road to Taking Control of Your Life, because the transformation is already occurring. You have taken the time to understand yourself. And you have used this resource called "you" to identify your missions in life.

You have launched the process of clearing away your irrational fears and putting your life into better balance by simplifying those areas in which you were once over committed. By making these improvements, you have made yourself a more finely-tuned resource, ready to realize your full potential.

Finally, like all truly successful people and organizations, you zeroed in on your single-most important mission in life—your PURPOSE. Then you supported it with a GOAL from each Area of Life. To further ensure the accomplishment of each GOAL, you identified a series of relevant ACTIONS complete with favorable conditions or times for putting them into effect.

YOU ARE NOW ON THE BRINK OF GETTING WHAT YOU WANT. You have, no doubt, already begun to see improvements in your life. Things are starting to go your way for a change. That's no coincidence! You are beginning to reap the benefits of being in control of your own life.

However, before you put this book on the shelf for a while, let's make sure that you get almost everything that you want. So get yourself ready to take the last few steps on your journey to happiness, health, wealth, and wisdom.

Step 6: Locking in YOUR PLAN

Okay, so you've got a PLAN and it's down on paper or maybe on computer disk. But how are you ever going to stay on track when you get back out there in the real world? All those demands and temptations will still be competing for your time and energy, just waiting to distract you.

It's probably not hard to imagine yourself in a situation like this: The kids want to go to the zoo. The VCR is out of commission and needs to be repaired. Your boss needs a project finished yesterday, and the TV commercials are reminding you it's time to buy a new car. Where will you get the time to put into action the things that you know are important to you and your future happiness?

The key is to take the time to LISTEN TO YOURSELF. I'm not talking about listening to yourself complain about being too busy to do the things you want to do. I'm not talking about hearing yourself moan that you will never experience your PURPOSE. I am talking about listening to yourself explaining

1   the traits and principles that are your strengths,

2   the importance of your Purpose,

3   the ways in which you are simplifying your life,

4   the importance of balancing your life, and

5   the GOALS and ACTIONS for each area of your life.

You need to spend time listening to these things which are vital to your future success and fulfillment, the things that will move you forward in your journey. If you don't, you will end up

● concentrating instead on ways other people want you to spend your time and energy,

● dwelling instead on the things you know are wrong with your life, and

● being stopped in your tracks or maybe even sliding backward.

To avoid this scenario, you must listen to yourself in ways that will keep you on track. It's as easy as reviewing and rereading your PURPOSE and PLANS periodically. An even more powerful tool is to record yourself on tape explaining who you are, why you are here, what you're going to do, and how you are going to do it.

This is the key to keeping yourself focused. Like any other tape, it will work on your subconscious and your conscious mind. The "B-Side" of the audio cassette you used as the Pathway to Your Subconscious to Identify Your Fears is just right for recording your Self-Talk Tape.

Listening to this tape periodically will help to "program your subconscious" with the elements of your PURPOSE and your Plans. Listening to this tape will bombard your subconscious with your message—not the messages of your parents, your spouse, your children, your boss, your friends, or the media. And your message is the ONLY message that is the road map to your future happiness. Listen to your own message first. It's the one you created, the one that will lead you where you want to go.

Some people prefer to get into a routine of playing their Self-Talk Tape regularly—perhaps weekly. About the only requirement is that you have 30 minutes to listen uninterrupted, preferably in a comfortable and relaxed position. It also helps to have some soothing background music recorded on the tape or playing while you listen.

Just remember, it's background music. Not too loud, not too much of a beat or rhythm that you get sidetracked. Just enough to help your message slide pleasantly into your mind.

Personally, I have found the best time to use my Self-Talk Tape is whenever I get frustrated or discouraged. Listening to the logic of my PLAN invariably puts things back into perspective for me and lifts my spirits. It also reminds me of several things I could be doing right now to Take Control of My Life and reduce these periods of unhappiness in the future.

Thirty minutes with your Self-Talk Tape will help change a self-pitying attitude of doom and gloom into a purposeful exuberance making you happy to be alive.

Don't throw away those written PLANS that you worked so hard to create! You will be working with them again in Chapter 9 to make sure that it all happens as you have planned. Equally important, record them on your Self-Talk Tape. Then listen to this tape frequently to KEEP Control of Your Life.

> "The human mind can discipline the body, can set goals for itself, can somehow comprehend its own potentiality and move resolutely forward." —Norman Cousins

Chapter 9

How to Make It All Happen
with
Scheduling and Monitoring

People who are happy and fulfilled spend more of their time doing the things

- they find most meaningful,

- in which they are most competent and

- that give them the most pleasure.

To make sure this happens, successful people, just like successful businesses, "rank order" their plans showing what they will do first, second, third, etc. Then, they establish schedules specifying <u>when</u> they will take each action. Finally, they monitor their progress to see <u>if</u> they are following through on their plans.

In this chapter, you will

- "rank order" your ACTION plans on MY PYRAMID OF PRIORITIES so you can overcome any temptation to <u>not</u> take action on the plans that support your GOALS and your PURPOSE.

- create MY LONG-TERM SCHEDULE so that you can focus on your most important ACTIONS. Then you can postpone the less meaningful ones while concentrating on the ACTIONS that will help ensure your happiness.

- construct MY WEEKLY SCHEDULE so you can show yourself that <u>you</u> (yes, YOU) have the power to move toward your GOALS and your PURPOSE while feeling the joy of doing what you want to do.

- monitor your progress so you can experience the satisfaction of realizing your dreams, the self-respect of being your own person and the exhilaration of fulfilling all of your potential.

During the process of taking these steps, you will create KEEPER #8—MY LONG-TERM SCHEDULE. If you have been worried up to this point that we were pulling your life apart, and trying to examine pieces which needed to be put back together, fret no more. Here is your opportunity to reassemble your life completely, with all the pieces fitting perfectly—just the way you designed it.

You will also build KEEPER #9—MY WEEKLY SCHEDULE. If you have been feeling overwhelmed at the thought of putting into motion all of the ACTION plans that you have identified, worry no longer. Here is your opportunity to break each ACTION down into manageable pieces so each step will be simple for you to perform. As you do this you will catch the rhythm that successful people use. Once you get the rhythm, YOU'VE GOT IT!

> "Do or do not.
> There is no try."
> —Yoda (Empire Strikes Back)

Now that you have:

- your resources defined,

- your missions identified,

- your excuses eliminated,

- your fears overcome,

- your life simplified and balanced,

- your purpose established,

- your goals set and

- your actions planned,

you are ALMOST in control. Your final tasks involve scheduling your ACTIONS and monitoring your progress. In other words, now that you know the "who," "why," "what," and "how" of your life, it's time to address the "when" and "if."

The Importance of Deciding WHEN to Take Action

Now you know what to do and how to do it, and your subconscious mind is helping you stay on track by using your Self-Talk Tape. But you still need to schedule your ACTIONS. Otherwise, all those good ideas might never jump off the page. If they stay glued to the paper, they will never help you advance on your journey of happiness and fulfillment.

I know it's incredibly easy to put things off—to let other demands take a higher priority than your own well-being. The way to combat this tendency to procrastinate is to nail down specific

ACTION items and schedule them. By deciding <u>when</u> to carry out one of your ACTIONS, you're committing yourself to making your plan a reality.

For example, the ACTION item on my PHYSICAL PLAN to join a health club could have remained right there on paper until long after my estate is settled. But, I took the final step of putting it on my schedule of "things that I am going to do." Successful people and businesses have learned the importance of the discipline created by making schedules and sticking to them. Now, let's get with the program and schedule <u>your</u> ACTION items.

What time frame works best for you? Don't know? Well, here's a suggestion. Try constructing two schedules:

1) MY LONG-TERM SCHEDULE. This timetable will contain

- items you expect to get to during the next three months,

- items that you plan to address within one year and

- a third group you hope to put into action sometime beyond the next year.

These ACTION items will make up KEEPER #8—MY LONG-TERM SCHEDULE.

2) MY WEEKLY SCHEDULE. This timetable (KEEPER #9) will concentrate solely on the items you plan to accomplish during the upcoming week.

Before you begin recording your ACTION plans on KEEPERS #8 and #9, you need to take one intermediate step. Think about it. You just came up with several ACTIONS suitable for each of the five Areas of Life. Which of these ACTIONS are the most important? Which should you do first?

Step 1: Prioritizing Your ACTIONS to Identify the Most Important

In order to schedule your ACTIONS, you first need to rank them—decide which are the most worthwhile and which can wait a while longer. Of course, such decisions are <u>not</u> cast in concrete. Deciding that something is relatively important now does not mean something else won't overtake it later. So, don't be afraid to make "mistakes"—you'll always have a chance to make adjustments later.

To help guide your thinking as you try to prioritize all these good ideas you have, I want you to construct a pyramid—MY PYRAMID OF PRIORITIES (see page 319). The pyramid will put a stop to your procrastination. At the top you will be staring at the most important ACTIONS you need to take in your life. The pyramid will also serve you well as you set about creating MY LONG-TERM SCHEDULE in the next step.

Right now you can start filling in the levels of the pyramid with the ACTIONS you've listed on KEEPER #7—MY (AREA OF LIFE) PLAN. As you review those five Plans, put them in the following order:

- first, the Area of Life in which you spend the least amount of time;

- second, the Area of Life in which you spend the next least amount of time; and

- so on, until you have all five Areas sequenced.

The Area of Life in which you spend the most amount of time will now be on the bottom. If you need to consult your KEEPER #5—MY WHEEL OF BALANCE, go ahead. This is one reason you created it. If you are at all like most of the people I work with, you probably have MY SPIRITUAL PLAN on top. Next would be MY PHYSICAL, MENTAL, and SOCIAL PLANS. MY CULTURAL PLAN would sit on the bottom. Your sequence will probably be very similar. This order will ensure that you review your ACTIONS by looking first at the Areas where you need to devote <u>more</u> time and energy. This procedure will help you achieve a balanced life.

Okay, of all the ACTIONS that you've written down on KEEPER #7, try to identify the ten most important. These ACTIONS concern your life in the near future (the next three months). Then enter them on the top tier of MY PYRAMID OF PRIORITIES. Why is each of these THE MOST IMPORTANT? You be the judge.

Perhaps,

- it is something you've wanted to do for a long time, or

- conditions are very favorable to do it right now, or

- it will help you make significant progress toward a goal, or

- it will help to bring your life into much better balance, or

- you will experience great satisfaction when you do it, or

- it will help you confront a primary fear head-on.

Whatever your reason or reasons, remember to include only the <u>ten</u> most important ACTIONS that you can take in the near future. As you transfer each to its place at the top of MY PYRAMID OF PRIORITIES, put a check next to that item on your Plan. That way, the next time you make a pass through your Plans, you won't have to consider that ACTION again.

"The more I want
to get something
done,
the less I call it
work."
—R. Bach

MY PYRAMID OF PRIORITIES

(Ordering my ACTION Plans)

1

2

3

4

5   6

7   8

9   10

First Tier
11   12   13

14   15   16

17   18   19

20   21   22

Second Tier
23   24   25   26

27   28   29   30

31   32   33   34

Third Tier
35   36   37   38   39

40   41   42   43   44

Now that the top of your Pyramid has been filled in, read through your Plans (KEEPER #7A-7E) a second time. Make sure you maintain the same sequence and identify the ten or so ACTIONS that you consider to be the next most important. As you transfer these items to the second tier of your Pyramid, remember to check them off your Plans as you go along.

After you repeat the procedure one more time filling in the third tier of your Pyramid, you will have prioritized as many as 34 ACTIONS. If there are any remaining items, list them at the bottom of your Pyramid. These items are possible future ACTIONS, but they have a low priority right now. Hopefully, this section will have a lot of Cultural ACTIONS—ones you may get around to someday when your life is more balanced than it is today.

Once again, congratulations! You have just taken another important step in the process of Taking Control of Your Life. You have allowed the "cream" of your ACTIONS to "rise to the top," where you can now "skim" them off and schedule them. And, just as significant, you have allowed the least important ACTIONS to sink to the bottom of your pyramid. You can ignore them for now. They'll be there waiting for you when you need them in the future.

Don't you feel good knowing that the most important things for you to do are now clearly identified? You will no longer be tempted to waste your time on ACTIONS that aren't meaningful to you. You have decided for yourself what ACTIONS are the most valuable as you create your own future—a purposeful life in which your ACTIONS support your GOALS which are helping you to fulfill your PURPOSE.

Step 2: Creating Your Long-Term Schedule to Focus Your Energy

KEEPER #8—MY LONG-TERM SCHEDULE is a natural outgrowth of MY PYRAMID OF PRIORITIES. This step involves transcribing ACTIONS from your Pyramid onto MY LONG-TERM SCHEDULE which consists of three time periods:

1) the next three months,

2) between three and twelve months, and

3) beyond twelve months.

These three periods correspond roughly with the top three tiers of MY PYRAMID OF PRIORITIES. I say "roughly" because, as you transcribe your highest priority ACTIONS to KEEPER #8 for the next three months, you need to examine each one again. Ask yourself: Is this something I can realistically accomplish in the next three months? If not, you should write it in the group of ACTIONS scheduled for completion between three and twelve months.

Otherwise, you may end up with a Long-Term Schedule that is overambitious and impossible to achieve. By questioning yourself on each item before writing it down, you have a much better chance of fashioning a reasonable schedule. A proper schedule will not burden you with guilt and frustration; it will motivate you with the trenchant zeal of a crusader.

As you move on to the transcription of the tier-two ACTIONS, you will need to examine the timing of each one similarly. Before placing any ACTION on MY LONG-TERM SCHEDULE as an item you will complete between three and twelve months, you should ask yourself the following two questions:

1   Is this item so important that I should try to accomplish it in the next three months? and

2   Should I be more realistic and postpone this item beyond twelve months?

If you said "yes" to either of these questions, your answer tells you where to transcribe it. Otherwise, enter the item in the grouping of ACTIONS that you will carry out between three and twelve months.

"Don't be afraid to take big steps.
You can't cross a chasm
in two small jumps."
—David Lloyd George

MY LONG-TERM SCHEDULE

(ACTIONS to be completed)

<u>During the Next Three Months:</u>

1.	5.	9.
2.	6.	10.
3.	7.	11.
4.	8.	12.

<u>Between Three and Twelve Months:</u>

1	5.	9.
2.	6.	10.
3.	7.	11.
4.	8.	12.

<u>Beyond Twelve Months:</u>

1.	6.	10.
2.	7.	12.
3.	8.	13.
4.	9.	14.
5.	10.	15.

The third section of Your Long-Term Schedule has room for ONLY 15 items. Be selective as you transcribe from MY PYRAMID OF PRIORITIES. Begin at the third tier and, if you have room, from the bottom tier. Don't belabor this last section. It is clearly the least important of the entire schedule. However, measure each item as you did above, in case one of these ACTIONS should be elevated to the group of items that you will undertake between three and twelve months.

Anyway, don't try to squeeze more ACTIONS onto MY LONG-TERM SCHEDULE than the form allows. Your Long-Term Schedule is intended to be ambitious but achievable. If you create it in that spirit, you will have a detailed road map for your future. This map will help you focus on the things that are most worthwhile to you. And, your map will help you act upon those things that are most important to the achievement of your GOALS and your PURPOSE.

Do you remember my client, "Jerry," who was unable to specialize—the one who wanted to keep all of his options open? It was the combination of his Pyramid and his Long-Term Schedule that finally enabled him to focus his energies. He overcame his fear of specialization. He is now a very successful marketer of Internet technology.

Think about it! MY LONG-TERM SCHEDULE is your unique creation. Yours alone!

- It expresses the traits and beliefs that make up your personality.

- It embodies the talents and principled roles that are your missions.

- It confronts the "gremlins" that you are in the process of overcoming.

- It includes your ideas for balancing and simplifying your life. And, MOST IMPORTANT,

- It represents the <u>implementation</u> of your ACTIONS which will let you achieve your GOALS and make it possible for you to **BE** the person who your PURPOSE says you are.

Can you feel it? <u>Your destination is in sight!</u> The rewards of taking control of your life are within reach. Fulfillment is almost within your grasp. Of course, you still need to perform—to actually do what you have laid out in MY LONG-TERM SCHEDULE. To help with this final step, you need to get into a weekly habit of listing what you are going to accomplish during the coming week.

Step 3: Creating Your Short-Term Schedule to Give You the Power

There's a saying that there are two types of people: those who make lists and those who work for people who make lists. I'm not sure who said it or why it happens that way, but I've certainly seen plenty of effective list-making in action.

A list is a way of focusing your attention on what is really important. A list helps you make sure that relevant matters don't get overlooked. It provides you with the motivation to get things done. It rewards you with satisfaction as you cross off completed tasks.

A good list has a life of its own. It is a living part of your existence. It also

- reminds you,

- prods you,

- fills in dead time for you,

- gives you a feeling of security that you are spending your time wisely, and

- gives you a sense of accomplishment when you cross off the last item, wad it up in a ball, and toss it into the "round file!"

Making a weekly list of the Tasks that you are going to complete will do all these things for you. When you throw away that list at the end of the week, you'll be thinking to yourself: "I not only stayed on top of my responsibilities and had fun this week, but also made some significant progress toward MY LONG-TERM SCHEDULE and my GOALS which support my PURPOSE. I am finally taking control of my life by advancing another step closer to being who I really am and having what I really want."

So, how do you go about listing things to do for the week? Perhaps you already do this. If so, you're familiar with the "magic" that lists possess and the ease of creating one. In addition to MY WEEKLY SCHEDULE on page 330, you'll find this important document in the KEEPER Forms Section as KEEPER #9.

It's not really a schedule in the sense that each Task has a time and day attached to it. It's more a list of Tasks that you should review each morning and again when you have free time. If you feel more comfortable specifying a particular time or day to perform each Task, there's room in the left-hand margin. Be cautioned, though. Such a strict schedule can apply added pressure you don't really need. A simple list is at least 90% as effective without sending you on a guilt trip for failing to deliver what you promised yourself at some exact time.

Speaking of "guilt," don't worry about being unable to complete <u>every</u> Task on your list. Things can and will happen during the week that you have no control over. That's okay. You can always start your list for next week with the items you couldn't finish.

You'll notice that there are two sections to KEEPER #9—MY WEEKLY SCHEDULE: a "will do" section and a "would like to do" section. Under "will do," list the Tasks to which you are willing to obligate yourself. Don't list the tasks you routinely do, such as going to class or doing laundry or going to the gym. Rather, enter here those occasional responsibilities or promises that you might forget if they aren't written on MY WEEKLY SCHEDULE.

For example, some of these "will do's" should be sub tasks of the ACTIONS on MY LONG-TERM SCHEDULE. Be sure to keep it handy when you are preparing your Weekly Schedule. For example, an ACTION that appeared on my "Next-Three-Month" Schedule at one point was <u>Join a Health Club</u>. As I began preparing MY WEEKLY SCHEDULE toward the end of that Three-month period, here are some sub tasks that began creeping onto my "will do" list on consecutive weeks:

- Week 1: Call some Health Clubs re: costs.

- Week 2: Visit Clubs to see facilities.

- Week 3: Ask about Trial Memberships at Clubs.

- Week 4: Make a decision re: Club Membership.

By completing these Tasks in a gradual and systematic way, I was able to break down the ACTION—Join a Health Club into doable Tasks. These tasks enabled me to accomplish the ACTION right on schedule without getting stressed out over some complicated and time-consuming project.

The "would like to do" section of MY WEEKLY SCHEDULE should be used similarly. Include here the preliminary steps or Tasks that will make completion of your ACTIONS easier and less stressful when the time is right. For example, I had Try Cross-Country Skiing as an ACTION I wanted to try in support of my Physical GOAL. Long before one of my kids expressed an interest in skiing, I included on my "would like to do" list such sub tasks as:

- Research at library alternative cross-country skiing locations.

- Write to locations for information.

- Call locations re: possibility of rental equipment.

These Tasks were not a high priority, but items on the "would like to do" list never are. These tasks are to be done on a time-available basis. Putting them on MY WEEKLY SCHEDULE is the first step to getting them done. Review your list each morning and again when you have free time. Be reminded of the importance of these tasks from time to time. You will be amazed at how much you can accomplish.

Part of the process of constructing MY WEEKLY SCHEDULE is to break down your ACTIONS into sub tasks. That way, you can accomplish things in a reasonable amount of time, and see real progress. The two examples above illustrate this point.

Just remember, you can't do it all in one week. Ask yourself: What shall I do first to carry out a specific ACTION? Then, what shall I do next? Each small step done in sequence will let you accomplish so much more than you have ever accomplished before. Why? Because you stay focused and committed to your ACTIONS, GOALS and PURPOSE.

> "The future belongs to those who prepare for it."
> —Malcolm X

MY WEEKLY SCHEDULE

(Tasks that I ......)

Will Do This Week:

1.
2.
3.
4.
5.
6.
7.
8.
9.

Would Like To Do This Week:

1.
2.
3.
4.
5.
6.
7.
8.
9.

You have now answered the question: When will I put my ACTIONS into, well, action? Your answers are contained in MY LONG-TERM SCHEDULE and MY WEEKLY SCHEDULE. *By sticking to these schedules, you are putting yourself in control of your own life.* Just you, no one else, will be in the driver's seat. You will begin enjoying the journey of life as you never have before. You will be doing what needs to be done so you can

- be who you really are and

- have what you really want.

There have been many steps along the way but each has produced benefits. By understanding who you are, you now have the self-confidence to be your own person. By removing the obstacles in your path, you have the freedom to be who you really are. And, by creating a plan for your future, you have a road map to follow leading to the life you want to live.

You have invested some of your valuable time in the process but the payoff is well worth it. You will live the rest of your life absorbing a great deal of success and happiness as you fulfill your PURPOSE.

Step 4: Monitoring Your Progress to Be All that You Can Be

To make sure you stay on track, you need to create a new schedule each week. Pick a time that's good for you and DO IT—each week. Maybe it's the first thing you do Monday morning or the last thing you do Sunday night. I personally find Sunday morning to be a most productive quiet time to construct my KEEPER #9—MY

WEEKLY SCHEDULE. But, whenever you do it, don't let a week go by without establishing your itinerary for the week. Although you have already devoted a lot of effort to be in control of your future, it is the self-discipline of your Weekly Schedule that will continue to make it happen!

It's okay if you didn't complete every "would like to do" item on last week's schedule. An item can be a "would like to do" for two or even three weeks before you get around to it. But, if time starts to get tight, putting the completion of an ACTION on MY LONG-TERM SCHEDULE in jeopardy, make sure you move the appropriate items off the "would like to do" list and onto your "will do" list.

For example, in order to Join a Health Club on schedule, I had to put the item "call some health clubs re: costs" on my "will do" list with just four weeks left on my timetable. Otherwise, I would have had to cram too much into those last four weeks when a lot of other things were going on as well.

Similarly, at the end of three months, you need to update KEEPER #8—MY LONG-TERM SCHEDULE. I hope you were realistic in creating your Long-Term Schedule and diligent about completing it. If you were, most of the ACTIONS you had planned to carry out are now behind you. If they are not, don't despair. I'm sure you made significant progress, and now have a better idea of what you can expect to accomplish while staying on top of all your ongoing duties and responsibilities.

Remember, the idea is not to try to do too much too fast. Instead, start to show some progress AWAY FROM a life in which you feel helpless and hopeless. Move TOWARD a life in which you experience the joy of being who you really are.

As you prepare subsequent MY LONG-TERM SCHEDULES, carry over any ACTIONS still in progress. Move them up the time scale to the empty slots created by your completed ACTIONS.

It's not necessary to go back to MY PYRAMID OF PRIORITIES every three months. However, do set priorities again once a year. You will be a year wiser, having learned how it feels to be in control. And, of course, things will have happened that you didn't expect.

Revising MY PYRAMID OF PRIORITIES annually will put you behind the wheel for another year of progress, success, and satisfaction. I have found that the best time for me to revisit my Pyramid is during my annual vacation:

- not the beginning of the vacation when the ongoing stresses of daily life are still fresh in my mind, and

- not in the middle of the vacation when I am totally enjoying the change of pace.

Instead, I work on MY PYRAMID OF PRIORITIES toward the end of my vacation. At that time, I have begun to put life back into perspective and the daily grind has yet to begin again.

Every few years, you'll want to go back to MY (AREA OF LIFE) PLANS. When you do, you will be amazed at the progress you have made—the number of ACTIONS you have actually made happen. Yes, you are in control! As you rethink your GOALS for each Area of Life, you will come up with new ACTIONS and the process will regenerate itself.

If you feel yourself slipping away from the planning process, remember all the tools you have created for yourself. These tools are for you to use during the rough times ahead:

- If you find you are doubting yourself, refer to KEEPER #6—MY PURPOSE WORKSHEET or listen to your Self-Talk Tape of your PURPOSE and also your GOALS and ACTIONS in each Area of Life.

- If you find yourself gravitating toward Cultural interests, update KEEPER #5—MY BALANCE WHEEL to see how bumpy your ride is becoming. This will remind you to keep your life simple and in balance.

- If old fears creep into your conscious mind, recite your Substitute Messages to put those negative thoughts in their place and review KEEPER #3—MY "DO SOMETHING" IDEAS to overcome your fears.

- If the ideas and expectations of others begin to overwhelm you, refer to KEEPER #1—MY RESOURCES and review who YOU really are. And,

- If you catch yourself going off on tangents, dust off KEEPER #2—MY MISSION STATEMENTS and remember why you are here.

You see? It's not difficult to be happy, healthy, wealthy and wise. You just have to know how. And now that you know how to take control of your life, you too, have the tools to join the ranks of those of us who enjoy happiness, good health, wealth and wisdom.

KEEPER Forms Section

KEEPER #1 — MY RESOURCES
     (The Highlights of My Personality)

KEEPER #2 — MY MISSION STATEMENTS

KEEPER #3 — MY "DO SOMETHING" IDEAS
     (To Confront My Fears)

KEEPER #4 — MY (AREA OF LIFE) ACTIVITIES

KEEPER #5 — MY WHEEL OF BALANCE

KEEPER #6 — MY PURPOSE WORKSHEET

KEEPER #7 — MY (AREA OF LIFE) PLAN

KEEPER #8 — MY LONG-TERM SCHEDULE
     (ACTIONS to be Completed)

KEEPER #9 — MY WEEKLY SCHEDULE

MY RESOURCES
The Highlights of My Personality

My character strengths (traits) are:

Creative   Supportive
Agreeable   Fair
Loyal   Strong
Responsible

My most significant limitations are:

Making Decisions
Communicating my thoughts

The activities I enjoy most are:

Reading   Self Care
Walking   Laughing
Parties   Play

The roles I prefer to play are:

Student   Artist
Teacher   Entrepreneur
Friend

My strongest institutional beliefs are:

Self Care / Responsibility
Metaphysics   Intuition
Exercise   alt Medicine

The most important principles that guide my life are:

Peace   Harmony
Clarity   Forgiveness
friendship   creativity   Service
Love   growth

MY MISSION STATEMENTS

****

Using my _____, I will be a
                    (traits and talents)

_____, guided by _____
      (role)   (principles)

for the benefit of _____.
                              (recipients)

****

Using my _____, I will be a
                    (traits and talents)

_____, guided by _____
      (role)   (principles)

for the benefit of _____
                              (recipients)

****

Using my _____, I will be a
                    (traits and talents)

_____, guided by _____
      (role)   (princilpes)

for the benefit of _____
                              (recipients)

****

MY MISSION STATEMENTS (cont)

****

Using my _____, I will be a
                    (traits and talents)

_____, guided by _____
        (role)   (principles)

for the benefit of _____ .
                              (recipients)

****

Using my _____, I will be a
                    (traits and talents)

_____, guided by _____
        (role)   (principles)

for the benefit of _____
                              (recipients)

****

Using my _____, I will be a
                    (traits and talents)

_____, guided by _____
        (role)   (princilpes)

for the benefit of _____
                              (recipients)

****

MY "DO SOMETHING" IDEAS
To Confront My Fears

****

To overcome my fear of _____, I could

_____ .
(possible course of action)

****

To overcome my fear of _____, I could

_____ .
(possible course of action)

****

To overcome my fear of _____, I could

_____ .
(possible course of action)

****

To overcome my fear of _____, I could

_____
(possible course of action)

****

MY "DO SOMETHING" IDEAS (cont)

****

To overcome my fear of _____, I could

_____

(possible course of action)

****

To overcome my fear of _____, I could

_____

(possible course of action)

****

To overcome my fear of _____, I could

_____

(possible course of action)

****

To overcome my fear of _____, I could

_____

(possible course of action)

****

To overcome my fear of _____, I could

_____

(possible course of action)

MY CULTURAL ACTIVITIES

Current	Ideas for Change
1. _____hrs	1. _____hrs
2. _____hrs	2. _____hrs
3. _____hrs	3. _____hrs
4. _____hrs	4. _____hrs
5. _____hrs	5. _____hrs
6. _____hrs	6. _____hrs
7. _____hrs	7. _____hrs
8. _____hrs	8. _____hrs

MY CULTURAL ACTIVITIES (cont.)

Current	Ideas for Change
9. _____hrs	9. _____hrs
10. _____hrs	10. _____hrs
11. _____hrs	11. _____hrs
12. _____hrs	12. _____hrs
13. _____hrs	13. _____hrs
14. _____hrs	14. _____hrs
15. _____hrs	15. _____hrs
16. _____hrs	16. _____hrs

TOTAL HOURS _____   TOTAL HOURS _____

% CULTURAL _____   % CULTURAL _____

MY MENTAL ACTIVITIES

Current	Ideas for Change
1. _____hrs	1. _____hrs
2. _____hrs	2. _____hrs
3. _____hrs	3. _____hrs
4. _____hrs	4. _____hrs
5. _____hrs	5. _____hrs
6. _____hrs	6. _____hrs
7. _____hrs	7. _____hrs

TOTAL HOURS _____   TOTAL HOURS_____

% MENTAL _____   % MENTAL _____

MY PHYSICAL ACTIVITIES

<u>Current</u>	<u>Ideas for Change</u>
1. _____hrs	1. _____hrs
2. _____hrs	2. _____hrs
3. _____hrs	3. _____hrs
4. _____hrs	4. _____hrs
5. _____hrs	5. _____hrs
6. _____hrs	6. _____hrs
7. _____hrs	7. _____hrs

TOTAL HOURS _____ TOTAL HOURS _____

% PHYSICAL _____ % PHYSICAL _____

MY SOCIAL ACTIVITIES

Current	Ideas for Change
1. _____hrs	1. _____hrs
2. _____hrs	2. _____hrs
3. _____hrs	3. _____hrs
4. _____hrs	4. _____hrs
5. _____hrs	5. _____hrs
6. _____hrs	6. _____hrs
7. _____hrs	7. _____hrs

TOTAL HOURS _____ TOTAL HOURS _____

% SOCIAL _____ % SOCIAL _____

MY SPIRITUAL ACTIVITIES

Current	Ideas for Change
1. _____hrs	1. _____hrs
2. _____hrs	2. _____hrs
3. _____hrs	3. _____hrs
4. _____hrs	4. _____hrs
5. _____hrs	5. _____hrs
6. _____hrs	6. _____hrs
7. _____hrs	7. _____hrs

TOTAL HOURS _____   TOTAL HOURS _____

% SPIRITUAL _____   % SPIRITUAL _____

MY WHEEL OF BALANCE

Percentage of Time Spent in Each Area of Life
(Before Changes)

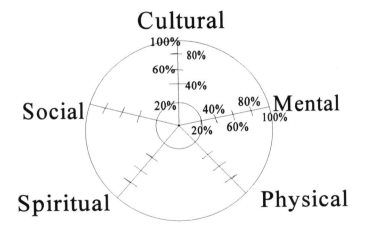

MY WHEEL OF BALANCE

Percentage of Time Spent in Each Area of Life
(After Changes)

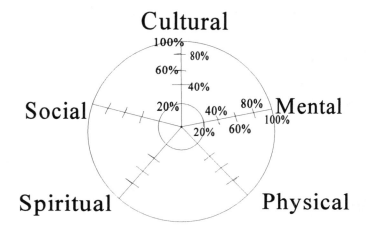

MY PURPOSE WORKSHEET

My Purpose in Life is to use my _____ to
(traits and talents)

be a _____ guided by _____,
(role) (principles)

for the benefit of _____.
(recipients)

	Goals	Actions
Physical		
Mental		
Social		
Spiritual		
Cultural		

MY PHYSICAL PLAN

<u>GOAL</u> -- (The target for my Physical life which will enable me to fulfill my PURPOSE):

_____

_____

_____

ACTIONS to consider	Comments
1.	
2.	
3.	
4.	
5.	
6.	
7.	
8.	
9.	
10.	
11.	
12.	
13.	
14.	

MY SPIRITUAL PLAN

<u>GOAL</u> -- (The target for my Spiritual life which will enable me to fulfill my PURPOSE):

_____

_____

_____

<u>ACTIONS</u> to consider	<u>Comments</u>
1.	
2.	
3.	
4.	
5.	
6.	
7.	
8.	
9.	
10.	
11.	
12.	
13.	
14.	

MY MENTAL PLAN

GOAL -- (The target for my Mental life which will enable me to fulfill my PURPOSE):

_____

_____

_____

ACTIONS to consider	Comments
1.	
2.	
3.	
4.	
5.	
6.	
7.	
8.	
9.	
10.	
11.	
12.	
13.	
14.	

MY SOCIAL PLAN

<u>GOAL</u> -- (The target for my Social life which will enable me to fulfill my PURPOSE):

_____

_____

_____

ACTIONS to consider	Comments
1.	
2.	
3.	
4.	
5.	
6.	
7.	
8.	
9.	
10.	
11.	
12.	
13.	
14.	

MY CULTURAL PLAN

<u>GOAL</u> -- (The target for my Cultural life which will enable me to fulfill my PURPOSE):

_____

_____

_____

<u>ACTIONS</u> to consider	<u>Comments</u>
1.	
2.	
3.	
4.	
5.	
6.	
7.	
8.	
9.	
10.	
11.	
12.	
13.	
14.	

MY LONG-TERM SCHEDULE
(ACTIONS to be completed)

During the Next Three Months:

1.	5.	9.
2.	6.	10.
3.	7.	11.
4.	8.	12.

Between Three and Twelve Months:

1	5.	9.
2.	6.	10.
3.	7.	11.
4.	8.	12.

Beyond Twelve Months:

1.	6.	10.
2.	7.	12.
3.	8.	13.
4.	9.	14.
5.	10.	15.

MY WEEKLY SCHEDULE
(Tasks that I ......)

<u>Will Do This Week:</u>

1.	
2.	
3.	
4.	
5.	
6.	
7.	
8.	
9.	

<u>Would Like To Do This Week:</u>

1.	
2.	
3.	
4.	
5.	
6.	
7.	
8.	
9.	

Appendix A

The Pathway to Your Subconscious
to
Identify Your Fears

The following message is meant to be personalized by you and then recorded on an audio cassette tape. The complete instuctions for this can be found in Chapter 4 of the book under Step 1 which begins on page 120. Everything that follows should be spoken into your tape recorder with the exception of the CAPITALIZED INSTRUCTIONS.

Find a comfortable sitting position. Close your eyes and relax. Now think about your breathing. As you slowly inhale, feel your stomach expand. As you exhale, breathe slowly, slowly, through your mouth. Continue breathing this way, focusing on the rising and falling of your stomach as you inhale....... exhale....... inhale....... exhale...... With each breath you are becoming more and more relaxed.

As you listen to the soothing music and breathe deeply, you can feel your feet and ankles relaxing. Now think of your legs, calves, and thighs and feel the tension drain away from them. As you think about relaxing your pelvic muscles, you find yourself sinking even more comfortably into your chair.

Next, allow your stomach and low back to relax. As you focus on the muscles in your upper back and chest, relax these parts of your body. Now concentrate on your shoulders and neck, allowing the tension to drain away. Let you arms and hands relax and feel heavy at your sides. And finally, relax the muscles in your face, particularly your jaw and forehead.

Your entire body is now free of tension. Your mind is open and receptive to good ideas. Imagine yourself in your ideal state without any limitations. Who are you as a person?

Think about your Eulogy (The Tribute to Your Life) ....
....(PAUSE 10 SECONDS).

What are you doing? Think about some of the roles you play in your Mission Statements ....(PAUSE 10 SECONDS).

What do you have? What people and possessions do you see around you? How do you feel? What good feeling do you have in this safe and ideal state of mind? ....(PAUSE 10 SECONDS).

As you listen to the soothing music in your state of total relaxation, breathing deeply and imagining your ideal self, consider this reason for your being here:

(RECITE YOUR FIRST MISSION STATEMENT) ....
....(PAUSE 15 SECONDS).

Consider this reason for your being here:
(RECITE YOUR SECOND MISSION STATEMENT) ....
....(PAUSE 15 SECONDS).

Consider this reason for your being here:
(RECITE AS MANY MISSION STATEMENTS AS YOU HAVE,
.............................PAUSING FOR 15 SECONDS AFTER EACH)

As you continue to relax and breathe deeply with the soothing music still playing, ask yourself: "what am I afraid of right now?" Don't try to question these fears or pass judgement on them. Just let them surface. Do you have any fears associated with your roles in each of the five areas of your life: Cultural ..... (PAUSE 5 SECONDS), Mental ..... (PAUSE 5 SECONDS), Physical ..... (PAUSE 5 SECONDS), Social ..... (PAUSE 5 SECONDS), and Spiritual ..... (PAUSE 10 SECONDS).

While the music continues to be a soothing influence on you, make a decision to do something about each of these problems. Repeat the following affirmation to yourself out loud: "I will confront each of my fears and excuses so that I may enjoy the freedom to be all that I can be"...(PAUSE 10 SECONDS).

Repeat this commitment to yourself 6 more times while maintaining your state of total relaxation: "I will confront each of my fears and excuses so that I may enjoy the freedom to be all that I can be"......
....(PAUSE 60 SECONDS).

Very shortly, I am going to count from 5 down to 1 and you will gradually become more and more alert. 5, you are more aware, 4, 3, you are more alert, 2, 1, you are fully awake and alert.

Annotated Bibliography

This Annotated Bibliography will help you decide what books are worth reading as you go about the process of taking control of your life. The topics are arranged alphabetically to help you find the material that you need. Most books are described from the standpoint of their

- Purpose and orientation,
- Major premise, and
- Potential value to you.

Only the most practical works have been included in this abridged bibliography. Some of the entries appear more than once if they are relevant to more than one topic.

TABLE OF CONTENTS

BRAINSTORMING

Ram Dass, <u>Journey of Awakening: A Meditator's Guidebook</u>, New York: Bantam, 1978. Cat-Brainstorming
A spiritual leader who has practiced a wide range of meditative traditions, Dass provides the reader with practical suggestions on how to find a personal meditative approach that works. He also includes an extensive list of groups that teach meditation.

Ann Faraday, <u>Dream Power</u>, Berkeley: Berkeley Publishers, 1973. Cat-Brainstorming
This is a comparison of several theories about dreams and their interpretations. It is cast in the context of information, albeit symbolic, that your brain produces which can be useful in your conscious thinking and decision-making.

Gail Sheehy, <u>Pathfinders: Overcoming the Crisis of Adult Life and Finding Your Own Path to Well-Being</u>, New York: William Morrow, 1981. Cat-Brainstorming
Sheehy's extensive research included 60,000 individuals who completed her Life History Questionnaire as she searched for "pathfinders." These are people who came through an adult passage or crisis in a creative and expanding way. They were unafraid of change and willing to take risks. Generalizing from these examples, she explains how anyone can become a pathfinder. As with her previous works, Sheehy cites many individual cases that may help you with your own brainstorming.

CAREER PLANNING

Richard Nelson Bolles, The 1994 What Color is Your Parachute, Berkeley: Ten Speed Press, 1994. Cat-Career Planning
An update of his original best seller from the 70's. Bolles leads the motivated reader through a series of personal exercises aimed at self understanding and a careful study of the world of work. The result is this practical manual for job-hunters and career-changers which can be used by young and old alike in their search for success and fulfillment at work.

Dean C. Dauw, Up Your Career, Palo Alto: Consulting Psychologist Press, 1980. Cat-Career Planning
Dauw prepared this large workbook for anyone, any age who is in the throes of a career decision. It starts out with Dr. John Holland's vocational approach and moves through other self-assessment procedures toward a tentative decision. There are special sections on the problems of women, the "mid-life crisis," how to choose a counselor, and employment agencies.

John L. Holland, Making Vocational Choices: A Theory of Careers, Palo Alto: Consulting Psychologists Press, 1973. Cat-Career Planning
This is an excellent summary of the research that resulted in Dr. Holland's Theory of Careers in which he relates six primary personality groupings to the occupational world. His pragmatic approach permits you to access your personality and then find compatible work situations that will maximize your career satisfaction.

John Loughary and Theresa Ripley, Career & Life Planning Guide, Palo Alto: Consulting Psychologist Press, 1976. Cat-Career Planning,

Cat2-Life Planning
Here is a useful workbook intended for adults who are dissatisfied with their current careers <u>and</u> are willing to consider change. You are lead through a realistic step-by-step process of analyzing your situation (assessing your needs, interests, and values), understanding the obstacles to change, and then implementing your decision.

Paul Stevens, <u>Stop Postponing the Rest of Your Life and Find Work Satisfaction (Achieving Career Satisfaction)</u>, Sydney: Center for Worklife Counseling, 1987. Cat-Career Planning
Stevens offers good discussions on such relevant topics as the mid-life crisis, burnout, life patterns and career life cycles. He believes that it is most important to analyze your past and build on both the good and the not-so-good. "You must find out who you really are today before taking charge of where you will be tomorrow".

U.S. Department of Labor, <u>Occupational Outlook Handbook</u>, Washington, D.C.: U. S. Government Printing Office, 1994. Cat-Career Planning
This Handbook describes what workers do, the education and training required, the advancement possibilities, the current employment outlook, the expected earnings and working conditions for several hundred occupations. Available in many libraries, it is a valuable resource for anyone making career decisions.

CLIMATE

W. S. Kals, <u>Your Health, Your Moods, and the Weather</u>, New York: Random House, 1982. Cat-Climate
This is a compilation of some convincing evidence that the weather

can have a dramatic effect on your behavior and your well being. Dr. Kals draws upon extensive research in showing the correlations that many people experience. There are also helpful suggestions on how to live more healthfully.

Helmut E. Landsberg, <u>Weather and Health: An Introduction to Biometeorology</u>, New York: Doubleday & Company, 1969. Cat-Climate
Understanding that each change in the weather requires an adaptation of the human mind and body, Dr. Landsberg explains how climatic conditions effect diseases as well as our moods and many of our psychological responses. After discussing the fairly obvious effects of wind, sun, and extreme cold, the author explains some of the more subtle influences such as electrical disturbances, barometric pressure changes, and the passage of cold fronts. Because on their effect on individual health and well-being, these climatic conditions also have an observable impact on group behavior.

FINANCE (PERSONAL)

Joe Dominguez and Vicki Robin, <u>Your Money or Your Life,</u>: Viking Penguin, 1992. Cat-Finances
In an attempt to put the financial side of life into perspective, the authors provide you with checklists, personal money questions, and formulas that are guaranteed to change your attitude toward finances.

Wanda Fullner, <u>A Primer on Personal Money Management-For Midlife and Older Women</u>, Washington, D.C., AARP, 1992. Cat-Finances
Despite the title, this primer is appropriate for men or women, young

or old. It takes you on a guided tour of fiscal responsibility starting with your goals and proceeding through record keeping, saving, credit, insurance, and where to get help. In workbook format, there are 19 separate steps with the suggestion that you construct and maintain a Financial Notebook containing all important information.

GENERAL BOOKS

Sharon B. Merriman and M. Carolyn Clark, <u>Lifelines: Patterns of Work, Love, and Learning in Adulthood</u>, San Francisco: Jossey-Bass, 1991. Cat-General
Based on a study of 400 people, the authors present their theory regarding the interactions between work, love, and learning in adult life. Practical tools and strategies are interspersed with many personal stories.

John-Roger and Peter McWilliams, <u>Life 101--Everything We Wish We Had Learned about Life in School But Didn't</u>, Los Angeles: Prelude Press, 1991. Cat-General
Based on the premise that "life is for doing, learning and enjoying," the authors provide perspective on such varied topics as religion, relationships, making mistakes, and bureaucracy. Their tools for making changes also establish a method, at least in theory, for enjoying life.

John W. Santrock, Ann M. Minett, and Barbara D. Campbell, <u>The Authoritative Guide to Self-Help Books</u>, New York: Guilford Press, 1994. Cat-General
Existing self-help books are categorized into sections such as: Adult Development, Self Fulfillment and Happiness, and Self Improvement

and Motivation. The entries are then rated on a scale of one to four stars based on a poll of professionals in the appropriate field. The best works are then described in some detail. This is a very comprehensive, current, and well written reference manual.

Alvin Toffler, <u>Future Shock</u>, New York: Random House, 1970. Cat-General
Rapid technological innovation in the industrial world is causing a psychological disorientation which is induced by change. Toffler believes that no one is sheltered from this phenomenon as it affects individuals, their relationships at work and their interpersonal relationships. If the rate of change continues to grow faster, individual adaptation will become increasingly difficult.

LIFE PLANNING

Richard Nelson Bolles, <u>The Three Boxes of Life and How to Get Out of Them</u>, Berkeley: Ten Speed Press, 1981. Cat-Life Planning
After debunking common myths with timely suggestions and perspective, Bolles applies his successful career planning techniques to making life changes in this practical (but sometimes tedious) manual. The tradition of dividing life into three parts--education, career, and retirement—bothers Bolles, so he proposes some enlightening alternatives for achieving a more compatible blend of study, work, and leisure.

Stephen R. Covey, <u>The Seven Habits of Highly Effective People: Restoring the Character Ethic</u>, New York: Simon & Schuster, 1990. Cat-Life Planning, Cat2-Choosing Success
Ben Franklin was an advocate of the Character Ethic in which

character traits and qualities form the foundation of success. Since World War II, we have adopted the Personality Ethic in which success results from our public image, our attitudes, our behavior, our skills and our abilities. Covey identifies seven habits and corresponding principles of effective people which encourages the resurrection of a principle-centered paradigm. His treatment of personal responsibility and interpersonal success are followed by very useful Application Suggestions.

Wayne W. Dyer, <u>Real Magic: Creating Miracles in Everyday Life</u>, New York: Harper, 1992. Cat-Life Planning
Dyer's work takes you on a spiritual path of purpose, magic, and meditation. He shows you how his philosophy of life can be applied successfully in your relationships, your finances, your personal identity, and your health.

Benjamin Franklin, <u>The Autobiography of Benjamin Franklin</u>, Kenneth Silverman, Ed., New York: Viking-Penguin, 1986. Cat-Life Planning
A jack-of-all-trades, master of many, Franklin was an accomplished printer, scientist, banker, merchant, soldier, patriot, philosopher, and statesman. His autobiography includes his formula for perfection or at least self improvement. After introducing the 13 virtues which he sought in his life, Franklin displays the "Log" he used to monitor his progress on a daily, weekly and quarterly basis.

Ken Keyes, Jr., <u>Handbook to Higher Consciousness</u>, Coos Bay, OR: Love Line Books, 1972-92. Cat-Life Planning
This is the premier publication documenting Keyes' Science of Happiness which involves loving everyone unconditionally. His 12 Pathways guide readers in the process of identifying, understanding, accepting, and reprogramming life addictions or habits.

Shad Helmstetter, Choices, New York: Pocket Books, 1990. Cat-Life Planning, Cat2-Self-Talk
This book is about deciding for yourself who you really want to be and what you really want from life. An advocate of the self-talk technique, Helmstetter sees everything in life as a personal choice. He includes a list of alternative choices in ten areas of life that can also be used as personal affirmations. There is a good balance of theoretical and practical considerations including several workbook pages for the reader to record personal decisions.

John Loughary and Theresa Ripley, Career & Life Planning Guide, Palo Alto: Consulting Psychologist Press, 1976. Cat-Career Planning, Cat2-Life Planning
Here is a useful workbook intended for adults who are dissatisfied with their current careers and are willing to consider change. You are lead through a realistic step-by-step process of analyzing your situation (assessing your needs, interests, and values), understanding the obstacles to change, and then implementing your decision.

Bradley C. McRae, Ed., Practical Time Management, Bellingham, WA: Self-Counsel Press, 1991. Cat-Life Planning
Rather than deal with time management in the work environment, McRae applies the same techniques to our personal lives. The explanations are comprehensive but succinct. Short exercises (19 in all) are provided to insure that the concepts will be applied to your life. Finally, the author includes forms to help guarantee that improvements made will remain permanent changes. Sample chapters include deciding what you want to do (brainstorming and goalsetting), monitoring your time, overcoming inertia, and managing your leisure time.

Nene O'Neill & George O'Neill, <u>Shifting Gears: Finding Security in a Changing World</u>, New York: M. Evans, 1974. Cat-Life Planning, Cat2-Choosing Success
The O'Neill's belief is that each of us has the potential and capacity for responsible self-determination. We can mold a personal future which provides a sense of fulfillment by expressing the creativity that is our very essence. They propose the development of a "life strategy" as the key to change. This book helps you in the task of "shifting gears" by leading, growing, understanding yourself, and accepting challenge. Chapters include: centering, decision-making, commitment, and self management.

M. Scott Peck, <u>The Road Less Travelled</u>, New York: Simon & Schuster, 1978. Cat-Life Planning
A practicing psychiatrist, Peck presents practical ways to confront life's problems using examples from his patients' histories. He emphasizes the construction of a "map of life" which is based on truth and a realistic view of life. Peck recommends that we ensure personal growth by constantly monitoring our maps and opening them for inspection through honest communication.

James Redfield and Carol Adrienne, <u>The Celestine Prophecy: An Experiential Guide</u>, New York: Warner Books, 1995. Cat-Life Planning
In this sequel to his best seller, Redfield reiterates his nine Insights regarding life and suggests exercises that readers should do to better understand themselves and their purpose. Meditation, help from others, and "trial decisions" are three methods that are advocated for making life changes.

John-Roger and Peter McWilliams, <u>Wealth 101</u>, Los Angeles: Prelude Press, 1992. Cat-Life Planning

Defining "wealth" in the broad sense as "contentment, joy, balance, equanimity, and inner peace," the authors use quotes from such sources as Miss Piggy, Douglas MacArthur, and Thoreau to put their ideas into perspective. The book helps readers discover their purpose and pursue their goals with dedication.

Gail Sheehy, <u>Passages: Predictable Crises of Adult Life</u>, New York: Bantam, 1977. Cat-Life Planning

Since Sheehy includes 115 case histories to illustrate her insights on the twenties, the thirties, the forties, and beyond, you will undoubtedly find several pages which seem to be describing your own situation. Some of her best sections describe: "A first solo flight," "What am I going to do with my life," "The couple puzzle," "Men's life patterns," "Women's life patterns," "The courage for a career change," "Where have all the children gone," and "The diverging sexual life cycles."

Gail Sheehy, <u>New Passages: Mapping Your Life Across Time</u>, New York: Random House, 1995. Cat-Life Planning

A mere generation after her first major publication, Sheehy's research has determined that there has been a revolution in the adult life cycle. This shifts all of the stages of adulthood ahead by 10 years. She has discovered a Second Adulthood beginning around the age of fifty when there is an exhilarating rebirth as people ask, "How shall we spend the rest of our lives?" Using essentially the same format as her original "Passages," Sheehy offers many case histories to illustrate: the flourishing forties, the flaming fifties, the serene sixties, and the sage seventies.

Barbara Sher, <u>Wishcraft: How to Get What You Really Want</u>, New York: Ballantine, 1986. Cat-Life Planning
Although her philosophy minimimizes the importance of understanding yourself, Sher focuses on a step-by-step approach to implementing your goals complete with charts and diagrams that produce concrete results.

Charles Spezzano, <u>What to Do Between Birth and Death: The Art of Growing Up</u>, New York: William Morrow, 1992. Cat-Life Planning
A practicing psychotherapist, Dr. Spezzano has a "folksie" writing style which makes this user's guide to adulthood very readable and practical. He helps you believe that <u>you</u> are the only one who can take responsibility for your life. His primary emphasis is on the issues involved in going from adolescence to adulthood: decision-making, marriage, families, money, power, and fame.

David Viscott, <u>Risking</u>, New York: Pocket Books, 1977. Cat-Life Planning
Self improvement involves taking risks. Uncertainty and danger are simply part of the process of reaching for a goal. This book is a guide to help you understand what happens when you take risks--including the feelings that you experience. Viscott tells you how to build the courage to take risks and discover a goal that is right for you. He also provides a good summary chapter of "Do's and Don'ts."

PHILOSOPHY OF LIFE

David L. Bender, <u>Constructing a Life Philosophy</u>, St Paul: Greenhaven Press, 1985. Cat-Philosophy of Life, Cat2-Spirituality
Bender includes an overview of the thinking of most religions

(Eastern and Western) as well as contributions of Franklin, Toynbee, Peck and Fromm.

Stephen R. Covey, A. Roger Merrill, and Rebecca R. Merrill, <u>First Things First: To Live, To Love, To Learn, To Leave a Legacy</u>, New York: Simon & Schuster, 1994. Cat-Self Understanding, Cat2-Philosophy of Life
As a followup to "7 Habits," Covey elaborates on one of the most important principles of successful people—personal management of your time and life. He emphasizes "relationships and results" instead of "time and things" as a means to balancing your life. Of course the first step to accomplishing anything worthwhile is to define what is really important. As such, the authors include three significant Appendices including: a Review of the Wisdom Literature (philosophy of life and self understanding) and an excellent Mission (in life) Statement Workshop for the reader.

Duane Elgin, <u>Voluntary Simplicity, An Ecological Lifestyle that Promotes Personal and Social Renewal</u>, New York: Bantam, 1982. Cat-Philosophy of Life, Cat2-Simplicity
The author advocates a balanced life in which we do not disperse our energy frivolously, but use our unique capabilities in ways that enhance the rest of our lives. Elgin provides a realistic perspective on such wide-ranging topics as historical civilizations, East-West philosophies, bureaucracies, consciousness, relationships and work.

Louis Gittner, <u>Listen, Listen, Listen</u>, Eastsound, WA: The Louis Foundation, 1981. Cat-Philosophy of Life
The 52 chapters (one for each week of the year) deal with contemporary problems and a successful approach to solving them. The book is designed to prompt readers into reaching their higher

self, and becoming involved with their true destiny. Although not focusing on specific problems, the lessons do reflect on the dangers of selfishness and rigidity from which all problems and maladies originate.

Ken Keyes, Jr., <u>How to Enjoy Your Life in Spite of It All</u>, Coos Bay, OR: Love Line Books, 1980. Cat-Philosophy of Life
This is a summary treatment of Keyes' philosophy that (1) you should love yourself and others, (2) you should convert your "addictions" to life preferences, and (3) your life is your teacher.

Ken Keyes, Jr., <u>Prescriptions for Happiness</u>, Coos Bay, OR: Love Line Books, 1981-93. Cat-Philosophy of Life
From Keyes' point of view, your happiness is assured if you (1) ask for but don't demand what you want, (2) accept whatever happens <u>now</u>, and (3) "turn up your love."

Hugh Prather, <u>Notes on How to Live in the World and Still Be Happy</u>, New York: Doubleday, 1986. Cat-Philosophy of Life, Cat2-Simplicity
Prather's philosophy of happiness involves practicing several principles such as living simply, in the here and now, with forgiveness, humor, concentration, and trust. He provides you with valuable perspectives on such topics as money, career, possessions, your body, and relationships.

John Marks Templeton, <u>Discovering the Laws of Life</u>, New York: Continuum, 1994. Cat-Philosophy of Life
Along the lines of Ben Franklin's <u>Poor Richard's Almanac</u>, Templeton spells out 200 basic laws of life arranged in 40 sections in his effort to help you in your "lifelong learning process".

Arnold Toynbee, Surviving the Future, Oxford: University Press, 1971. Cat-Philosophy of Life, Cat2-Simplicity
This authority on the history of civilizations shares his philosophy that we should live for loving, understanding, and creating even if it means self-sacrifice. By contrasting animals with humans, Toynbee provides perspective on the importance of self understanding and education.

RELATIONSHIPS

Eric Berne, Games People Play, New York: Grove Press, 1961. Cat-Self Understanding, Cat2-Relationships
Berne explains his Transactional Analysis in both theory and practice. On the personal level, this book can help you understand the effects of different motives, the way motives interact, and the power of self-fulfilling prophecies. On the interpersonal level, Berne documents some of the classic two-person "games" that we play in relationships.

Dale Carnegie, How to Win Friends and Influence People, New York: Pocket Books, 1982. Cat-Relationships
Before preparing one of the first self-help books of its kind, Dale Carnegie did extensive research into the nature of successful relationships. He identifies numerous principles or practical suggestions that were true in 1936, when this work was first published, and still apply today. These are easy-to-use techniques that are expected to make you a better friend.

Thomas A. Harris, I'm OK - You're OK, New York: Harper & Row, 1969. Cat-Relationships
Continuing to develop Transactional Analysis, Dr. Harris outlines the

system of "script" writing between parents and children. He offers insight into how we develop the Parent, Child, and Adult in ourselves through our relationships with others. Because of Harris' many examples, you will likely find your own predicament explained in some detail along with the message, "If you don't like the trap, you can change it."

Ken Keyes, Jr., <u>The Power of Unconditional Love</u>, Coos Bay, OR: Love Line Books, 1990. Cat-Relationships
This is Keyes' perspective on relationships in which he offers 21 guidelines for beginning, improving, and changing your most meaningful relationships.

David Lewis, <u>The Secret Language of Success: Using Body Language to Get What You Want</u>, New York: Carroll & Graf, 1989. Cat-Relationships
Only seven percent of meaning is contained in spoken words. Most communication takes place non-verbally: appearance, posture, gesture, gaze, and expression. Lewis proposes 31 basic rules as a practical guide to using body language at work and at play for achieving greater social success.

Virginia Satir, <u>People-Making</u>, Palo Alto: Consulting Psychologist Press, 1972. Cat-Relationships
This is a nontechnical discussion of Satir's perspective on families (health, welfare, and survival). It is written in a basic, fast-paced style appropriate for both layman and professional. From this book you will gain new insights about your familial relationships.

William C. Schutz, <u>The Interpersonal Underworld (FIRO)</u>, Palo Alto: Science and Behavior Books, 1970. Cat-Relationships

This is Dr. Schutz's account of his three-dimensional theory of personality whose basic dimensions are the interpersonal needs of inclusion, control, and affection. Measured in terms of both behavior and feelings, these scales are able to assess both desired feelings and expressed feelings. FIRO is particularly relevant to the compatibility of relationships as well as self-assessment.

SELF UNDERSTANDING

Eric Berne, Games People Play, New York: Grove Press, 1961. Cat-Self Understanding, Cat2-Relationships
Berne explains his Transactional Analysis in both theory and practice. On the personal level, this book can help you understand the effects of different motives, the way motives interact, and the power of self-fulfilling prophecies. On the interpersonal level Berne documents some of the classic two-person "games" that we play in relationships.

Lucia Capacchione, The Creative Journal: The Art of Finding Yourself, Athens, Ohio: Swallow Press, 1994. Cat-Self Understanding
Taking the approach that nothing works better than a journal for exploring your innermost thoughts and feeling, Capacchione has developed over 50 exercises in journal keeping. Although simple, the exercises stimulate self-assessment, confidence building, planning and goal achievement. There is also a good mix of verbal expression and graphic art.

Stephen R. Covey, A. Roger Merrill, and Rebecca R. Merrill, First Things First: To Live, To Love, To Learn, To Leave a Legacy, New York: Simon & Schuster, 1994. Cat-Self Understanding, Cat2-

Philosophy of Life
As a followup to "7 Habits," Covey elaborates on one of the most important principles of successful people—personal management of your time and life. He emphasizes "relationships and results" instead of "time and things" as a means to balancing your life. Of course the first step to accomplishing anything worthwhile is to define what is really important. As such, the authors include three significant Appendices including: a Review of the Wisdom Literature (philosophy of life and self understanding) and an excellent Mission (in life) Statement Workshop for the reader.

David Keirsey and Marilyn Bates, Please Understand Me-Character and Temperament Types, Del Mar, CA, Gnosology Books, 1984. Cat-Self Understanding
After providing you with a short 70-question personality inventory of the Myers-Briggs type, the authors explain a simple self-scoring procedure. Armed with the knowledge of your personality type (one of the 16 possible), you are then given an entertaining and useful description of each type. There are also special chapters on the compatibility of each type with regard to childhood, mating, and leadership.

Isabel Briggs Myers with Peter B. Myers, Gifts Differing, Palo Alto: Consulting Psychologist Press, 1980. Cat-Self Understanding
The authors explain the many subtleties in the behavior of the 16 personality types identified by the MBTI (Myers-Briggs Type Indicator) Personality Inventory. After reviewing the theory of Carl Jung and its embellishments, they carefully describe each personality type. There are also chapters devoted to the compatibility of types with regard to marriage, learning environment, and career.

Virginia Satir, <u>Your Many Faces</u>, Palo Alto: Consulting Psychologist Press, 1978. Cat-Self Understanding

Satir believes that everyone is unique based on the many "faces" they have, such as fear, love, anger and joy. She guides you on a pleasant exploration of self understanding <u>and</u> self-acceptance.

SELF-TALK

Frank Caprio and Joseph R. Berger, <u>Helping Yourself with Self-Hypnosis: A Modern Guide to Self-improvement and Successful Living</u>, Englewood Cliffs, NJ: Prentice-Hall, 1963. Cat-Self-Talk

Based on the premise that self-suggestion is the most important aspect of self-improvement, the authors advocate hypnosis which relies on the relationship between the conscious and the subconscious mind. Since hypnotic suggestions bypass the conscious mind, they are an important form of self-suggestion that work for many people. After explaining in detail how to achieve self-hypnosis, Caprio and Berger offer many practical affirmations that will cover most aspects of your personal life.

Harry Hazel, <u>The Art of Talking to Yourself and Others</u>, Kansas City: Sheed & Ward, 1987. Cat-Self-Talk

You are constantly talking to yourself, and what you say is extremely important in terms of shaping your self image, being successful, and getting along with others. Reprogramming habits that have been built up over the years takes at least six weeks of consistently positive self-talk. Meditation is the best way to accomplish this. Hazel also provides an excellent perspective on relationships including the compatibility of different types of people.

Shad Helmstetter, <u>Choices</u>, New York: Pocket Books, 1990. Cat-Life Planning, Cat2-Self-Talk

This book is about deciding for yourself who you really want to be and what you really want from life. An advocate of the self-talk technique, Helmstetter sees <u>everything</u> in life as a personal choice. He includes a list of alternative choices in ten areas of life that can also be used as personal affirmations. There is a good balance of theoretical and practical considerations including several workbook pages for the reader to record personal decisions.

Shad Helmstetter, <u>What to Say When You Talk to Yourself</u>, New York: Pocket Books, 1986 Cat-Self-Talk

According to Helmstetter, our brains get "programmed" by everything we hear from the world around us <u>and</u> from our own Self-Talk (everything we say when we talk to ourselves). Since we live out our lives by acting on the programs that are the strongest, he explains how to use this very powerful planning technique, Self-Talk.

<u>SIMPLICITY</u>

Duane Elgin, <u>Voluntary Simplicity, An Ecological Lifestyle that Promotes Personal and Social Renewal</u>, New York: Bantam, 1982. Cat-Philosophy of Life, Cat2-Simplicity

The author advocates a balanced life in which we do not disperse our energy frivolously, but use our unique capabilities in ways that enhance the rest of our lives. Elgin provides a realistic perspective on such wide-ranging topics as historical civilizations, East-West philosophies, bureaucracies, consciousness, relationships and work.

Arthur Gish, <u>Beyond the Rat Race</u>, Scottdale, PA: Herals Press, 1973. Cat-Simplicity
Here is an examination of the nature and relevance of living simply from a Christian point of view. Gish includes discussions on spending less and enjoying more, simplicity as a lifestyle, and the cost of affluence.

Hugh Prather, <u>Notes on How to Live in the World and Still Be Happy</u>, New York: Doubleday, 1986. Cat-Philosophy of Life, Cat2-Simplicity
Prather's philosophy of happiness involves practicing several principles such as living simply, in the here and now, with forgiveness, humor, concentration, and trust. He provides you with valuable perspectives on such topics as money, career, possessions, your body, and relationships.

Arnold Toynbee, <u>Surviving the Future</u>, Oxford: University Press, 1971. Cat-Philosophy of Life, Cat2-Simplicity
This authority on the history of civilizations shares his philosophy that we should live for loving, understanding, and creating even if it means self-sacrifice. By contrasting animals with humans, Toynbee provides perspective on the importance of self understanding and education.

SPIRITUALITY

David L. Bender, <u>Constructing a Life Philosophy</u>, St Paul: Greenhaven Press, 1985. Cat-Philosophy of Life, Cat2-Spirituality
Bender includes an overview of the thinking of most religions (East and West) as well as contributions of Franklin, Toynbee, Peck and Fromm.

Jonas Salk, <u>Anatomy of Reality--Merging of Intuition and Reason</u>, Washington, D.C.:College & University Personnel Association, 1983. Cat-Spirituality
In the words of the renown scientist, Dr. Salk, "human beings have a feeling, sensitivity, and understanding for where they are in the cosmos and in the world, in time as well as in space. It is this feeling and understanding that link us to our historical and evolutionary past and future." He concludes that the merging of intuition and reason will provide wisdom for the resolution of the personal, societal, global, and cosmic struggles that we encounter.

Huston Smith, <u>The Religions of Man</u>, New York: Harper and Row, 1958. Cat-Spirituality
The premier work providing an overview of the major religions of the world. Smith explains the primary characteristics of: Hinduism, Buddhism, Christianity, Taoism, Islam, Judaism, and Confucianism.

Charles T. Tart, ed., <u>Transpersonal Psychologies</u>, New York: Routledge, 1975. Cat-Spirituality
Eight experts in various spiritual disciplines present their "religions" as psychologies. Included are Zen, Visuddhimagga, Yoga, Gurdjieff, Arica, Sufi, Christian mysticism, and Western Magick. There is also an interesting chapter by Tart on Orthodox Western Psychology.

STRESS

Peter G. Hanson, <u>The Joys of Stress</u>, New York: Andrews, McMeel, & Parker, 1985. Cat-Stress
This work puts stress into perspective by helping you identify your own level of stress. Hanson emphasizes the problems with too little as well as too much stress. His approach to stress management

involves finding a balance in life among financial sufficiency, personal happiness, sound health, and respect on the job. There are excellent illustrations and highlights here of key ideas and suggestions.

Christine Maslach, Burnout-The Cost of Caring, Palo Alto: Consulting Psychologist Press, 1982. Cat-Stress
Written with the primary helping professions in mind, Maslach's findings apply similarly to any service occupation. They are all susceptible to the stresses that cause burnout. Illustrated with many examples, the book describes the burnout syndrome, its causes and effects and suggests ways of dealing with it or even preventing it.

Hans Selye, Stress without Distress, New York: Signet, 1974. Cat-Stress
Widely recognized as the foremost medical authority on stress, Selye discovered the biological connection between persistent tension and the weakening of the human organism. This book explains his prescription for mobilizing stress for creative purposes and enjoying a full life in harmony with nature.

Dennis Shea and Kristen Barber, Stress and the Power Nap, Acton, MA: Copley Publications, 1993. Cat-Stress
Since taking a nap is just an extension of relaxing, a common stress reducer, Dr. Shea reasons that a power nap (taken for 20 or 30 minutes in mid-afternoon) is for people seriously interested in controlling stress in their lives. Billed as "The Book Designed to Put You to Sleep", this work is a lighthearted but serious treatment of an often overlooked stress reduction technique.

SUCCESS

Les Brown, <u>Live Your Dreams</u>, New York: William Morrow, 1992.
Cat-Choosing Success
This highly acclaimed speaker has written an excellent motivational
document based on his own experiences. It is particularly strong in
the areas of choosing success and setting goals.

Stephen R. Covey, <u>The Seven Habits of Highly Effective People:
Restoring the Character Ethic</u>, New York: Simon & Schuster, 1990.
Cat-Life Planning, Cat2-Choosing Success
Ben Franklin was an advocate of the Character Ethic in which
character traits and qualities form the foundation of success. Since
World War II, we have adopted the Personality Ethic in which
success results from our public image, our attitudes, our behavior, our
skills and our abilities. Covey identifies seven habits and
corresponding principles of effective people which encourages the
resurrection of a principle-centered paradigm. His treatment of
personal responsibility and interpersonal success are followed by very
useful Application Suggestions.

Wayne W. Dyer, <u>Your Erroneous Zones</u>, New York: Funk &
Wagnalls, 1976. Cat-Choosing Success
"It's your life; do with it want <u>you</u> want" Dyer urges in his chapter
which encourages the reader to "take charge of yourself." To help
with this process, Dyer identifies many common examples of self-
defeating behavior, and offers suggestions for change. Frequently
shared barriers to self-improvement are: preoccupation with the past,
worrying about the future, expecting justice, and procrastination.

Nene O'Neill & George O'Neill, <u>Shifting Gears: Finding Security in a Changing World</u>, New York: M. Evans, 1974. Cat-Life Planning, Cat2-Choosing Success
The O'Neill's belief is that each of us has the potential and capacity for responsible self-determination. We can mold a personal future which provides a sense of fulfillment by expressing the creativity that is our very essence. They propose the development of a "life strategy" as the key to change. This book helps you in the task of "shifting gears" by leading, growing, understanding yourself, and accepting challenge. Chapters include: centering, decision-making, commitment, and self management.

Penelope Russianoff, <u>When Am I Going to Be Happy? How to Break the Emotional Bad Habits That Make You Miserable</u>, New York: Bantam Books, 1988. Cat-Choosing Success
Here you will find practical suggestions on how to break free from emotional ruts. Russianoff offers tools like the "broken record" technique for assertiveness training and the "statute of limitations" technique to conquer depression.

Index

A

Actions, 199-205, 208-11, 221-24
    Area of Life Plans, 225-28
    Purpose Worksheet, 219
Activities, 158-60
    in Areas of Life, 165-70, 182-84, 335
    Worksheet, 160-65
Affirmations, 100, 142-46, 185, 360
American Motors, 207-08, 215
Annotated Bibliography, 24, 361-86
Areas of Life, 90, 93, 96-98, 148, 156-59, 199-201, 218-222
    allocation of time to, 172-175, 195
    cultural, 93, 95, 165-270, 186-93, 287-307
    mental, 91, 260-71
    Plans, 225-28
    physical, 91, 229-46
    social, 92, 273-85
    spiritual, 92, 247-58
    symbols for, 91-93
Author's messages
    afterward, 394-95
    foreword, 8-9

B

Bach, R. (quote), 318
Balance, 21, 148
    achieving, 150, 183-84
    importance of, 41-45, 90, 150-55
    measuring, 172-75
    Wheel of, 43, 155-58, 334
Beliefs, 68, 69, 71, 94
    system of, 251-54
Book evaluation, 396-97
Borrowing, 300-01
Brainstorming, 241-42, 362-363
Browning, Dr. Iben, 236
Burnout, 13, 153-54, 170
    See also Stress
Byrne, Robert (quote), 201

C

Career
    change, 188, 294
    compatibility, 287-94
    planning, 288-94, 362-66
    selection, 287, 294
Change, 17, 20, 60-61, 149, 175, 179, 211
    at work, 265-67

Jonson, Ben (quote), 272

K

KEEPER Forms, 23, 55, 78,
    83, 101, 114, 121, 135,
    158, 194, 211, 335-357
Keller, Helen (quote), 286
Kelley, Walt (quote), 192

L

Leno, Jay, 59
Life planning, 362, 368-73
Life Planning Institute, 1-2,
    394-98
Life's work
    see Purpose
Lists, 325-28

M

Marketable skills, 93, 151,
    192
McWilliams, Peter, 367, 371
    (quote), 87
Meditation, 99-100, 241, 257,
    270, 305
Melatonin, 235
Meyer, Paul J. (quotes), 74,
    184

Mission, 33-34, 82, 85, 94
    statements, 83, 88, 90, 96,
    100-08, 121-22, 150,
    214-16, 334-35
    workbook, 86
    worksheet, 97-99
    vs. purpose, 213
Money, 22, 294
    borrowing, 300-01
    consumer credit, 300
    saving, 296-97
    spending, 300-02
    See also Finance
Monitoring, 312-14, 331-34

O

Oppenheim, James (quote),
    155
Order form, 396
Organization, 45-46

P

Patino, Rick (quote), 164
PAS
    see Personality Analysis
    System
Pasteur, Louis (quote), 257
Peale, Norman Vincent
    (quote), 221
Personality, 55-58, 94, 263-
    265

Afterward

Because of my positive personal experience with the Life Planning Process, I am very excited to hear about the improvements that you have realized. On the next page you will find a Book Evaluation Form that I encourage you to use to record your adventure with the process. Thanks for forwarding it to me in care of Life Planning Institute.

Life Planning Institute also offers workshops and seminars dealing with the various Parts of the Book. Some people find a group environment helpful in taking their steps toward happiness, good health, wealth and wisdom. Please inquire regarding plans for future group workshops.

Since other people prefer individual assistance with the steps of the Life Planing Process, you too may want to hire a personal "coach." Please contact the Life Planning Institute to explore how you can be "coached" through the steps you need to take to enjoy the happiness, success and fulfillment shared by others.

A personal coach can help you map out the "right plan" for your future. You can be sure that the path you and your coach define will reflect who you are and why you are here. This will ensure that you have the self-confidence to actually carry out your plan and make it come true.

You can also be sure that the future you design will include positive ways to overcome any debilitating fears or complexities that you may be harboring. Resolving these roadblocks will energize you by giving you the freedom and the time to live the life you want to live.

Finally, you and your coach will identify a roadmap for you to follow that supports your purpose in life: goals and actions that are important to your physical, mental, social, spiritual and cultural well-being. Putting these things down on paper will give you the peace of mind and self-respect that comes with taking control of your own life. Carrying out these plans will generate the feelings of power and joy that accompany a life of happiness, good health, wealth and wisdom.

Also available from Life Planning Institute are supplementary computer software packages to help you with specific concerns such as career planning, stress reduction and relationship problem-solving. You will find on the Order Form, additional software designed by Drew Software International, developers of the Personality Analysis System (PAS) Shareware Program that accompanied this book. The full-blown PAS includes the capability to determine whether or not specific jobs fit your personality. Using it with others also makes it a valuable communications tool for any relationship you are in or may be contemplating. The PAS+ (Advanced PAS) is also able to identify areas of stress or potential stress in your relationships. The Team or Family Section helps you understand the basis for compatibility and sources of conflict among team/family members.

Once again, thank you for allowing me to share with you the secrets that I have discovered: the steps to a happy, healthy, wealthy and wise future. I am so sure that you will find this book to be a valuable asset that I am offering a 30-day money-back guarantee.

Kent McArthur

Book Evaluation Form

<u>Features:</u> I believe the book helped me to

- ☐ Understand myself better
- ☐ Simplify my life
- ☐ Identify my purpose in life
- ☐ Achieve my goals
- ☐ Stay focused & motivated
- ☐ Overcome my fears
- ☐ Balance my life
- ☐ Make a plan
- ☐ Schedule action plans
- ☐ Take control of my life

<u>Benefits:</u> Please record the benefits that you experienced by using the book and the Life Planning Process.

- ☐ Self-esteem
- ☐ Self-direction
- ☐ Self-actualization
- ☐ Freedom
- ☐ Reduced stress
- ☐ Fulfillment
- ☐ Spiritual growth
- ☐ Improved health
- ☐ Synchronicity
- ☐ Inner Peace
- ☐ Self-confidence
- ☐ Self-control
- ☐ Self-respect
- ☐ Happiness
- ☐ Love
- ☐ Balance
- ☐ Comfort
- ☐ Liberation
- ☐ Structure
- ☐ Joy of living
- ☐ Self-understanding
- ☐ Self-motivation
- ☐ Security
- ☐ Job satisfaction
- ☐ Hope
- ☐ Contentment
- ☐ Success
- ☐ Focus
- ☐ Wisdom
- ☐ Wealth

This book definitely improved the quality of my life by _____

_____

_____

_____

_____

The most important thing this book did for me was _____

_____

_____

_____

_____

<u>Steps of the Life Planning Process:</u>

Were any of the steps difficult for you? Please indicate.

☐ Taking the computerized Personality Test,
☐ Learning the five Areas of Life,
☐ Communicating with my subconscious,
☐ Distinguishing my fears from excuses for not taking action,
☐ Determining how to confront my fears,
☐ Deciding how to simplify my life,
☐ Identifying my purpose in life,
☐ Distinguishing between goals and action plans,
☐ Prioritizing my action plans,
☐ Recording my self-talk tape.

The book failed to live up to my expectations because _____
_____
_____
_____
_____

The next edition of the book should definitely include _____
_____
_____
_____
_____

Please return a copy of your evaluation form to the publisher:

Life Planning Institute
P.O. Box 415
Rathdrum, ID 83858

Or, email your comments to: evaluation@HappyForLife.com

Order Form

Photocopy or Return this Form with payment to:

Life Planning Institute, Inc.
P.O. Box 415
Rathdrum, ID 83858
1-888-216-1846

Or visit our Website: HappyForLife.com

Please send _____ copies of the book HOW TO BE HAPPY, HEALTHY, WEALTHY & WISE: The Guide to Taking Control of Your Life @ $24.95	$
PAS (Personality Analysis System): This family version also shows whether specific jobs match your personality @ $90 each.	$
PAS+ (Advanced PAS): Includes evaluation of personal stress and interpersonal compatibility & conflict with others @ $495 each.	$
Special Combination Packages:	
PAS and one copy of the Book @ $99	$
PAS + and one copy of the Book @ $499	$
Every five copies of the Book @ $99	$
Coaching by Life Planning Institute: (Includes Book) @ $249	$
Shipping & Handling*	$
Idaho Residents add 5% Sales Tax	$
TOTAL	$

* For S&H: add $3.50 for 1st book and $.75 for each additional book.

Name_____ Tel.# _____

Address _____

Organization:_____

☐ VISA   ☐ M/C   #_____

Expiration Date_____ Signature ___ _____

Order Form

Photocopy or Return this Form with payment to:
Life Planning Institute, Inc.
P.O. Box 415
Rathdrum, ID 83858
1-888-216-1846
Or visit our Website: HappyForLife.com

Please send _____ copies of the book HOW TO BE HAPPY, HEALTHY, WEALTHY & WISE: The Guide to Taking Control of Your Life @ $24.95	$
PAS (Personality Analysis System): This family version also shows whether specific jobs match your personality @ $90 each.	$
PAS+ (Advanced PAS): Includes evaluation of personal stress and interpersonal compatibility & conflict with others @ $495 each.	$
Special Combination Packages:	
PAS and one copy of the Book @ $99	$
PAS + and one copy of the Book @ $499	$
Every five copies of the Book @ $99	$
Coaching by Life Planning Institute: (Includes Book) @ $249	$
Shipping & Handling*	$
Idaho Residents add 5% Sales Tax	$
TOTAL	$

* For S&H: add $3.50 for 1st book and $.75 for each additional book.

Name_____Tel.# _____
Address _____
Organization:_____
☐ VISA   ☐ M/C   #_____

Expiration Date_____ Signature _____

Notes